MRI Primer

MRI
Primer

William Oldendorf, M.D.
and
William Oldendorf, Jr.

Raven Press New York

Raven Press, Ltd., 1185 Avenue of the Americas, New York, New York 10036

Made in the United States of America

Library of Congress Cataloging-in-Publication Data

Oldendorf, William H. (William Henry), 1925–
    MRI primer / William Oldendorf and William Oldendorf, Jr.
      p.   cm.
    Includes bibliographical references and index.
    ISBN 0-88167-769-8
    1. Magnetic resonance imaging. I. Oldendorf, William.
II. Oldendorf, William H. (William Henry), 1925–   Basics of
magnetic resonance imaging. III. Title.
    [DNLM: 1. Magnetic Resonance Imaging. 2. Nuclear Magnetic
Resonance. WN 445 044b]
RC78.7.N83043 1991
616.07′548—dc20
DNLM/DLC
for Library of Congress   91-12340
                                                        CIP

9 8 7 6 5 4 3 2 1

To Stella Z.

Contents

Preface   ix

A Note on Symbols and Abbreviations   xi

Acknowledgments   xiii

1   Introduction: Diagnostic Probes   1

2   Magnetic Resonance: A Familiar Example   9

3   Nuclear Magnetic Resonance   15

4   Imaging   23

5   Tissue Characterization: T_1 and T_2 41

6   Tissue Characterization and Pulse-Sequencing   69

7   The MRI Scanner   117

8   Sample MRI Scans   151

9   Advantages and Limitations of MRI   165

10 Advantages and Limitations of CT   183

11 Future of MRI   195

Appendix: An Introduction to Quantum Process   201
in MRI

Bibliography   213

Subject Index   215

Preface

MRI Primer is written as an introduction to the field for non-experts and is not intended as an extensive text on MRI. We present here a simple exposition of certain aspects of MRI that are important to understand in order to be able to use this valuable diagnostic tool intelligently in a clinical setting. The basic principles are presented nonmathematically, using no equations and a minimum of symbols and abbreviations. For those requiring a deeper understanding of MRI, this book will help facilitate the transition to standard texts.

MRI Primer provides readers with two levels of introduction to this subject. Those who desire an overview of the field can read Chapters 1 through 5 and 7 through 11, skipping the more technical Chapter 6 and Appendix. Those who would like a more in-depth introduction to the principles of MRI should include Chapter 6 and the Appendix. This additional material will also prepare readers for standard texts on the subject.

In summary, Chapters 1 through 5 present a general introduction to the phenomenon of nuclear magnetic resonance and how it is used in imaging. Chapter 1 introduces the concept of diagnostic probes, stressing x-rays (used in radiography and CT) and magnetic fields (used in MRI). Chapter 2 discusses magnetic resonance, using a compass needle as an example. In Chapter 3, the transition to the magnetic resonance of the atomic nucleus is made. Chapter 4 describes the principles of imaging. In Chapter 5, the terms T_1 and T_2 are defined, and their relationship to tissue characterization presented. Also, the fundamental role of thermal magnetic noise in T_1 and T_2 is discussed.

Chapter 6 introduces the magnetization vector as a convenient means of expressing nuclear behavior. T_1 and T_2 are described in more depth, and their role in imaging presented. The spin-echo pulse-sequence and the relationships of T_1 and T_2 to image brightness are introduced.

Chapter 7 describes the basic hardware components of an MRI scanner, including the design of the main magnet and gradient coils. Chapter 8 presents sample MRI scans, illustrating how MRI characterizes tissue. Chapters 9 and 10 review MRI and CT, respectively. Limitations and advantages of each imaging technique are discussed, and the two techniques compared. Some clinical correlates of MRI relaxation processes (T_1 and T_2) are presented. Chapter 11 speculates on future directions of this versatile clinical probe.

The Appendix provides a brief introduction to the quantum processes in MRI.

William Oldendorf
William Oldendorf, Jr.

A Note on Symbols and Abbreviations

The physical process upon which MRI is based—nuclear magnetic resonance (NMR)—was recognized in 1946. For the next 30 years it was used largely as a chemical analytical tool, under the name NMR. Consequently, the first scanners to exploit nuclear magnetic resonance to produce medical images were termed *NMR scanners*.

However, the use of the word "nuclear" caused concern among patients, who associated nuclear with radioactive, although there is no radioactivity or indeed any ionizing radiation involved. As a result, the term MRI (magnetic resonance imaging) came into use, although some confusion still exists about the use of these terms. In this book, NMR refers to the basic phenomenon of nuclear magnetic resonance (and to its use in chemical analysis in a laboratory setting); MRI refers to the process that exploits the physical phenomenon of NMR to make medical images in a clinical setting.

The basic physical phenomenon of NMR is easily demonstrated, but its application to MRI is more complex. Although the crude phenomenon can be detected with very simple equipment, to fully exploit its many ramifications requires an elaborate theory and complicated equipment.

As in most scientific specialties, the traditional NMR literature assigns many abbreviations or symbols to various aspects of the process. An excellent book published in 1971 (Farrar and Becker) lists 127 such abbreviations. Although many of these represent simple units, most refer to complex phenomena. To aid the reader's introduction to this field, we have used a nonmathematical approach, choosing to use no symbols or abbreviations except CT, NMR, MRI, T_1, and T_2.

Acknowledgments

Writing an introductory text on a complex subject is a difficult task which would not have been possible without the help of two people: Leon D. Braun, the artist who produced the many detailed illustrations that accompany this text, and Nancy Goldsmith-Rose, the editor whose knowledge of both science and language helped clarify the presentation of the text.

We would also like to thank Amy L. Annis for copyediting and proofreading assistance and the many colleagues who have generously offered their time to answer questions. We are especially indebted to Drs. Ray Gangarosa (Picker International), Frank Anet, Donald Fredkin, and William G. Bradley.

As always, many thanks are due to Stella Z. Oldendorf for long hours of material assistance and moral support.

William Oldendorf
William Oldendorf, Jr.

MRI Primer

1

Introduction: Diagnostic Probes

The physician confronted by a sick patient needs to know the nature of the malfunction and often is starved for information that might lead to a diagnosis. Our eyes see only the surface; what we wish to examine is the body's interior. To acquire this information, the physician interrogates the patient's body by means of various probes. Each probe interacts in some way with the tissues; the nature and extent of the interaction and its anatomic location are noted.

Classical physical diagnosis is the art of using little or no artificial apparatus to learn about the properties of living tissue. It uses the simplest probe—the palpating finger—which moves over the surface of the patient, interrogating such features as skin texture or subsurface masses. Limited access to the inside of the body may be gained through examination of its orifices, but this provides information only about structures near the orifice. Using only the senses of touch and position, the physician performs the simplest form of clinical image reconstruction: imagination. The sensory input from the fingers is used to form, in the mind, an image of the interior of the body. The physician's imagination, enriched by training and experience, makes this technique surprisingly accurate. A skilled surgeon examining the abdomen can, by feeling for internal organs and listening to their sounds, produce a remarkably informative image of the unseen abdominal organs.

In modern terms, the physician is using a sequence of instructions (a mental algorithm) by which the image is constructed in the mind from the simple palpation (input data). Although the probe needed for imaging by palpation is inexpensive and portable, this technique provides only limited information and is restricted to only a few accessible anatomical regions.

In another of the common probing procedures, percussion, the fingers of one hand are placed on the surface of the body, and the fingers of the other hand are struck against them. This creates a new probe, the advancing compression wave front (sound) that passes into the body. Over the chest, a certain quality of thump is heard, and over the abdomen, another. The character of the sound is determined by the shape and size of gas-filled cavities in the chest or intestine. Audible resonances in the gas in these regions are evoked by the input of sound energy, and they are heard and interpreted by the physician. Using a knowledge of the general internal anatomy and what commonly goes wrong with it, the physician is able to form in the mind, a crude image of likely internal abnormalities.

In magnetic resonance imaging (MRI) an analogous process of percussion is carried out. Instead of being percussed for audible resonances in gas-filled cavities, the body is percussed magnetically for magnetic resonances, which are then analyzed. MRI can be thought of as magnetic percussion.

While simple manual percussion can provide only limited information about the tissues, it can often be of use in patient management. Its limited information value is balanced by its great simplicity and by the absence of any apparatus other than the physician's hands (the transmitter), ears (the receiver), and brain (the computer), which together serve to construct an image of the body's internal condition.

MODERN PROBES

Much of the progress in diagnostic research has been directed to the development of more versatile probes. The first of these probes was the X-ray, discovered by Roentgen in 1895. To varying degrees, X-rays penetrate all visually opaque objects, their freedom of passage varying according to the nature of the object.

Roentgen's first subject was a hand, which he placed over a photographic plate, so that the X-rays cast a shadow of its bones. Because the X-rays from early sources were weak (by modern standards) they could penetrate only a short distance through tissues; as a consequence, the relatively thin hand was a favorite early subject for demonstration. Nonetheless, Roentgen had provided the physician with access to the interior of the living body, beyond the reach of existing probes. This advance was nearly as revolutionary as the first anatomical dissection had been, several centuries earlier.

Although they are enormously valuable, there is evidence of an impending decline in the use of X-rays in clinical diagnosis. Newer probes that are more informative are appearing. Just as palpation is useful but limited in scope, simple shadow images using X-rays are useful but are unable to provide direct images of the soft tissues, where most disease arises.

THE INTRODUCTION OF CT

Until 1972, ordinary medical radiographic films were made using essentially the same apparatus and techniques of a half-century earlier. In 1972, EMI Ltd., of England, made public the prototype of an apparatus that has been recognized as the most significant development in the clinical use of X-rays since their discovery by Roentgen: the computerized tomographic (CT) scanner.

This new development was a complete departure from classical radiography, which had used a wide shower of X-rays to cast shadows of body parts on a photographic film. In 1967, Godfrey N. Hounsfield, an EMI computer engineer, began applying a computer to the problem of reconstructing cross-sectional images of the body from information gathered by a narrow beam of X-rays. The beam entered the edge of the cross-section of the body being imaged. After traversing the body, the emerging X-rays were counted and the number lost in passage through the body was calculated. The position of the beam was changed many times in the course of the scan, so that any one cross-section of the body was examined many times from many directions. A computer, properly instructed, reconstructed the density (specific gravity) of the tissue in the cross-section being examined. The resulting CT scan could be thought of as though the cross-section had been cut from the body, placed on a radiographic plate, exposed, and the resulting film developed and viewed on a viewbox much as an ordinary radiograph (Figure 1–1).

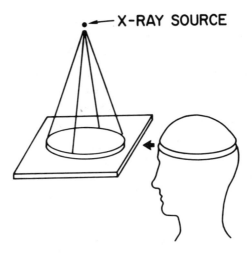

FIG. 1–1. An image comparable to a CT scan could be made by freezing the body, sawing out a slab of tissue, placing the slab on an X-ray plate, and making a radiograph of it. CT accomplishes the same process using a beam of X-rays, which enters the slice from its edge and traverses the entire slice. The image is then reconstructed by a computer.

CT and related diagnostic imaging methods provide so much three-dimensional structural detail that the scan cannot be displayed as if the body were being viewed from an external point (as in standard radiography). If this were done, the structures would be superimposed on each other, and the information would be incomprehensible. It would be as though one were attempting to examine the contents of a book that had been specially constructed with transparent cover and pages so that only the type was visible. With the book closed, the words and letters of the text would be superimposed, and, even if the book were just a few pages thick, only a meaningless jumble would be visible. The solution is to open the book and look at one page at a time. Each time we open a book and view the exposed pages individually, we perform tomography on the book (Figure 1–2). Similarly, in the body, we must slice it up (perform tomography) and look at one slice at a time.

CT scanning was immediately recognized as revolutionary, and subsequent experience has confirmed this first impression. The earliest images, which were exclusively of brain, were crude by mod-

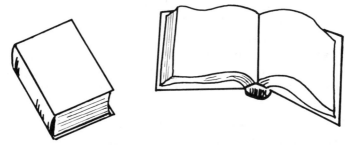

FIG. 1–2. A closed book could not be read, even if the pages and cover were transparent, because the words would all be superimposed. Opening the book isolates a page, allowing its detail to be seen. This is equivalent to performing tomography. The wealth of detail provided by modern imaging techniques requires the image to be displayed tomographically.

ern standards, but showed pathology clearly enough to indicate that CT would be a quantum leap forward in medical diagnosis. Among many other honors, Hounsfield received the Nobel prize for this work in 1979.

CT scanning allowed a limited but repeatable view of living brain structure. Such a view of brain structure had previously been available only after death, when the brain could be removed and chemically fixed to make it firm enough to be cut mechanically into sections. CT allowed what was, in essence, a limited autopsy during life. Because it was painless and essentially harmless, CT could be employed at even the faintest suspicion of early brain disease. And, unlike the diagnostic tests available to that time, it could be repeated freely to follow the course of a disease. As a result, many non-fatal diseases were accessible to scrutiny for the first time. Fatal diseases were visualized throughout their courses and not just at their terminal stages. Although we emphasize imaging of the head in this book, almost any region of the body could be used as an example.

Today, X-ray CT has become as vital to the practice of neurology and neurosurgery as radiography of the skeleton is to orthopedic surgery. Our knowledge of cerebrovascular disease has been greatly advanced and many traditional beliefs, which were based on observation of the clinical course and subsequent autopsy (perhaps years after the disease began), have been completely changed. Management of brain tumors was greatly facilitated, since they were recognized accurately at much earlier stages of development. The acute management of head trauma has been greatly advanced. Brain atrophy in many degenerative diseases can now be measured harmlessly and with more accuracy than at autopsy. In many elderly patients, considerable atrophy is seen, often without significant brain dysfunction.

Many other examples could be given of the major impact that CT scanning has had on diagnostic medicine; its effect can be summed up as revolutionary. By 1985 there were approximately 7,000 CT scanners worldwide, about one-third each in Japan and the United States, and the remaining one-third in other countries. With this resounding success story, why is CT application leveling off? Development of newer, more advanced CT scanners has nearly ceased and sales have leveled off, mostly representing replacement of older machines that are no longer state-of-the-art. Part of the reason for this decline is the limited tissue characterization offered by CT. Because the extent to which X-rays interact with tissue is proportional to the density of tissue, a CT scan is a map of specific gravity. With injection of contrast media, we see a superimposed distribution of iodine, but these two sources of information are all that are offered by CT scanning (see Chapter 10). Much of the declining interest in CT scanning is due to the appearance of a much more sophisticated diagnostic probe: the magnetic field.

THE MAGNETIC PROBE

The subject of this book is magnetic resonance imaging (MRI), the technology that utilizes this highly versatile probe. The interaction of magnetic fields and tissue atoms is so elaborate that much more information can be obtained than with X-rays. New strategies are constantly being developed so that tissue characterization has improved dramatically over the past few years, and there is every reason to believe that the field will continue to develop for many years to come. Just as there are many more moves and strategies in the game of chess than there are in checkers, the tissue interaction available in MRI potentially offers very much more tissue characterization than is possible with CT.

THE DECLINING AUTOPSY

There have been so many advances in clinical imaging techniques in recent years that the postmortem examination is becoming obsolete. This is not in itself a cause for concern, however, since it should be the indirect purpose of all diagnostic research to make the traditional autopsy unnecessary. During the past century, the autopsy has been considered the ultimate standard of diagnosis. This remains true today, but the role of the autopsy is waning. In major teaching centers, only about one-fourth as many autopsies are performed as there were two decades ago. There are several factors contributing to this, such as the desire for cost containment and the refusal of most health insurance companies to pay for them. But a major factor is that fewer "curiosity autopsies" are now performed. Before modern imaging, patients often died with no clear diagnosis ever having been made; the cause of death was clarified only at autopsy. With modern diagnostic methods, this happens much less often, and a plausible diagnosis is usually arrived at during life. Modern imaging methods play a large role in arriving at this diagnosis.

Although the autopsy is a superb diagnostic and teaching process, it has severe limitations and disadvantages. The person being autopsied cannot benefit from the procedure. Usually, only fatal disease processes are seen, and only in their terminal state; non-fatal diseases are seen only coincidentally. Since the autopsy may be performed several days after death, postmortem artifacts are prominent; these are superimposed on the often-prolonged dying process, which may have created its own artifacts. The results of the autopsy are largely anatomical; only limited chemical studies are possible. The disturbances in function that were the source of patient complaints during life may only be inferred.

Although X-ray CT did much to improve the accuracy of clinical diagnosis, its limitations are now being realized. MRI supplies a wealth of information, exceeding CT in most instances. It promises a giant step toward the "pre-mortem autopsy" that we so urgently seek, since, while there is life, there is hope of benefitting the patient under study.

Still, the autopsy will not completely disappear for a very long time. So much information has been accumulated by pathologists, that the vast data bank of traditional histology will remain the gold standard for many decades to come.

2

Magnetic Resonance:
A Familiar Example

Magnetic resonance is one of the interactions between a magnet and a magnetic field. The most familiar magnet is a compass needle. The most familiar magnetic field is that of the earth. The most familiar interaction of a magnet with a magnetic field is the alignment of a compass needle with the earth's field: the compass points north and south. By studying the interaction of a compass needle and the earth's magnetic field, we can gain important insights into the principles of magnetic resonance imaging.

If we start with a compass needle at rest, pointing north, and then tap one tip of the needle with our finger, the needle first deflects away from north but is then drawn back toward its original northerly orientation. It overshoots north, and continues in a to-and-fro oscillatory movement. Gradually, the oscillatory movement diminishes until all of the energy the needle received from our finger is lost to mechanical friction and air drag. The compass again comes to rest pointing north (Figure 2–1). The frequency of this oscillatory movement is the needle's *natural frequency*, which depends both on the characteristics of the compass needle—its dimensions, strength of magnetization, and mass—and on the strength of the external field. This last point is worth repeating: the natural frequency is proportional to the external field strength. In a stronger magnetic field, the compass needle oscillates faster: for example, if the external field strength doubles, the natural frequency doubles.

The magnetic field of the earth is not uniform over its entire surface. The field converges at the north and south magnetic poles and spreads out over the surface of the earth in between. Near the poles,

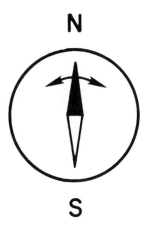

FIG. 2–1. A compass needle aligns itself north and south in the earth's magnetic field. If deflected from its north-south heading, it oscillates at a frequency proportional to the local magnetic field strength.

the earth's field is strongest, being about 0.7 gauss (the gauss is a common unit of magnetic field strength) and, at the equator, weakest, about 0.3 gauss. Between the equator and poles, there is a gradual transition in field strength (Figure 2–2A). Such a gradual change in field strength between one location and another is called a *magnetic field gradient*, or simply a *gradient*, a term that will be used often in this book.

We could make a compass that oscillates at a natural frequency of one cycle per second at the equator. If we travelled north from the equator with the compass, we would find the frequency of oscillation changing gradually: the farther north, the higher the frequency of oscillation. At the North Pole, the compass would oscillate about 2.3 cycles per second because the earth's field is 2.3 times stronger there. If it were properly calibrated, the compass needle could be used as a crude navigational device, using natural frequency to estimate latitude (Figure 2–2B).

In this simple example, we have the essential elements of MRI:

1. A compass needle, when placed in a magnetic field, aligns itself with the field.

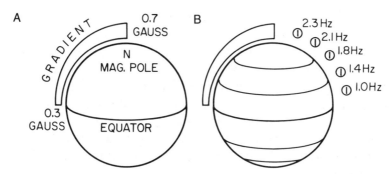

FIG. 2–2. A: The earth's magnetic field is not uniform. Since it converges on the poles, the field strength there is greater than at the equator. The gradually rising field strength between equator and poles constitutes a magnetic field gradient. **B:** A compass oscillates faster near the pole. Properly calibrated, it could be used as a crude navigational device, to determine latitude from frequency of oscillation.

2. When stimulated, the compass needle oscillates at a frequency proportional to the strength of the magnetic field.

3. In a gradient magnetic field that varies in strength in a known manner, the location of the compass needle can be deduced from its frequency of oscillation.

We further note that this process includes a means of stimulation (our finger) and a means of detecting the movement (our eye).

ALTERNATIVE MEANS OF
STIMULATION AND DETECTION

We could also develop other means of stimulating the compass needle and observing its subsequent behavior. (Extending the analogy in this manner will allow us to better explain magnetic imaging of tissues in later chapters.)

Stimulation by an Alternating Source

In the above example, we stimulated the compass needle by a single strong tap of our finger. If instead we apply a series of very light taps, evenly spaced, the compass needle would again absorb energy and be deflected from true north. But if we change the frequency of the tapping, by making the time interval between taps longer or shorter, we would observe an interesting phenomenon: At one particular frequency, the compass would absorb energy most efficiently (and be deflected away from north by the largest angle). At other frequencies, the compass needle would absorb energy less efficiently, and would be deflected away from north by a much smaller angle. The specific frequency of tapping at which the most efficient absorption of energy occurs is the natural frequency of the compass needle.

Another example of applying energy at a particular frequency is to be found in pushing a child on a playground swing. After a single push, the swing moves to-and-fro at its natural frequency. To sustain the swinging motion, we apply a series of pushes, which we intuitively time to correspond to the natural frequency. Like the compass needle, the swing can most efficiently absorb the energy when our pushes are applied at this frequency. Attempting to push at other frequencies would be less efficient.

Resonance

This is the phenomenon of *resonance*: the compass needle absorbs energy most efficiently from an external alternating source when the frequency of the alternating source matches the natural (resonant) frequency of the compass needle.

Resonance is a general phenomenon in which an object most efficiently absorbs energy from an external, alternating energy source. In the case of a compass needle, the resonant frequency is determined by the length and mass of the needle, how strongly magnetized it is, and the strength of the external field it is in. (In general, the term *resonant frequency* will be used in this book instead of *natural frequency*. The subtle distinction is that natural frequency is used to describe oscillation of an object after it has been energized by a single, brief stimulation, while resonant frequency usually refers to the rate of oscillation of an object exposed to a continuous alternating source of energy.)

INSTRUMENTATION OF
STIMULATION AND DETECTION

If we wished to remotely stimulate the compass needle, rather than tap it physically we could place a small coil of wire adjacent to one tip of the needle. Passing brief pulses of current through this coil creates a magnetic field proportional to the current, thus imparting brief magnetic "kicks" to the needle. A series of magnetic kicks would transmit energy to the compass needle in the same way as tapping with our finger. Again, if we varied the frequency of the magnetic pulses, the amplitude of swing would be greatest at the resonant frequency.

Similarly, if we were unable to observe the movement of the compass needle visually (or required greater accuracy), we could electronically instrument the compass-based navigational device. The simplest means of measuring the oscillatory movement of the compass needle after stimulation would be to place near it a coil of wire that would act as an antenna. Since the needle is itself a magnet, its movement would induce voltage in the coil. Its oscillatory frequency could be measured if the induced voltage were amplified and sent to an electronic frequency analyzer. By this means, a simple number (its frequency) could indicate the latitude of the compass without the compass actually being viewed.

The phenomenon of resonance pervades science. It governs the exchange of energy between fingers and guitar strings, between earthquake shocks and buildings, between passing trains and rattling windows, between wind and swaying bridges, and even between atomic nuclei.

3

Nuclear Magnetic Resonance

The behavior of compass needles in the earth's magnetic field was introduced in Chapter 2 to present the concept of magnetic resonance. A compass needle is actually a small bar magnet that oscillates at a particular frequency when driven from its resting state. The frequency of its oscillation is proportional to the field strength in which it finds itself. While the simplest means of stimulating a compass needle is by a simple tap of the finger, it can also be driven from its resting state by subjecting it to an alternating external magnetic field. When the frequency of alternation occurs at the needle's natural or resonant frequency, the compass needle absorbs energy most efficiently.

We are interested in the magnetic properties of living tissues, which contain no compass needles. But there are small magnets with some of the properties of a compass needle: the nuclei of certain atoms.

MAGNETIC NUCLEI

Among the elements having magnetic nuclei, hydrogen is of the greatest biological interest, both because it has the most highly magnetic nucleus and because it makes up two-thirds of the atoms in living tissues. In MRI, it is largely the hydrogen in tissue water that is imaged.

Since the hydrogen nucleus is the simplest of all nuclei, consisting of only a single proton, imaging of hydrogen is often referred to as *proton imaging*. This can be misleading because other nuclei, which are more complex, also contain protons; but in imaging terminology, these are identified by the chemical name of the atom, such as phosphorus or fluorine. In this book, therefore, *hydrogen nucleus* is used instead of *proton*.

Why should the nuclei of some atoms be magnetic? We have seen how a permanent magnet such as a compass needle or bar magnet produces a surrounding magnetic field (Figure 3–1A) Magnetic fields are always created by the movement of electrical charges, either positive or negative. This is true even in a permanent magnet, where the field is produced by orbiting electrons locked into the crystalline structure of the magnet. When a current of electrons (negative charges) passes through a piece of straight wire, a magnetic field surrounds the wire. If we bend the wire into a circular loop, a magnetic field similar to that of a bar magnet is created (Figure 3–1B).

For our purposes, we may consider that the nucleus of the hydrogen atom is a very small volume of space containing a positive electrical charge. Due to two properties of the hydrogen nucleus, the electrical charge creates a magnetic field analogous to that produced by a loop of wire carrying moving charges. One of these properties is that the positive charge is located at some distance

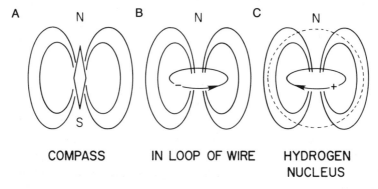

COMPASS   IN LOOP OF WIRE   HYDROGEN
                                       NUCLEUS

FIG. 3–1. A: A compass needle is an example of a permanent magnet. **B:** Magnetic field produced by electric current in a loop of wire is an example of electromagnetism. **C:** In the hydrogen nucleus, movement of electric charge also creates magnetic field. The positive charge is located off center, somewhere within the volume of the nucleus. Because the nucleus is spinning about an axis, the moving charge behaves like the current in the loop of wire, producing a magnetic field. This is nuclear magnetism.

away from the center of the nucleus; the other is a property called *spin*. The term *spin*, as used in classical physics, refers to the rotation of an object about an axis. When used in nuclear physics, spin describes a roughly analogous phenomenon. Spin is an inherent property of all fundamental atomic particles and, like nuclear mass, does not change.

We can think of the hydrogen nucleus as physically spinning about an axis, but unlike familiar spinning objects in the real world, its rate of rotation is unknown and it does not slow down due to friction. Its positive charge is not located at the exact center of the nucleus but is located some distance from the axis, so that, as the nucleus spins, the positive charge revolves in an approximately circular path, much as an electron in a loop or wire. This movement of the positive charge produces a magnetic field (Figure 3–1C).

There are about 1800 recognized combinations of protons and neutrons; each of these combinations is called a *nuclide*. Most of these are unstable (radioactive). Of the approximately 280 stable nuclei, about 100 are magnetic. The rule of thumb for determining whether a nucleus is magnetic is described in Figure 3–2.

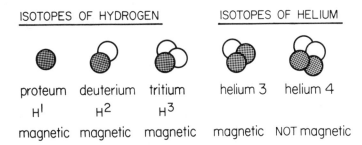

FIG. 3–2. A nucleus is some combination of protons and neutrons; when it contains either an unpaired proton or neutron, or both, it has a net spin and is therefore magnetic. The five simplest nuclei are shown, the protons black and the neutrons white. A pair of protons or a pair of neutrons have opposed spins that cancel each other (as in helium 4). To be magnetic, a nucleus must have an unpaired proton (as in all three isotopes of hydrogen) or an unpaired neutron (as in helium 3) or one of each (as in deuterium).

PROPERTIES OF A MAGNETIC NUCLEUS

The compass needle and hydrogen nucleus are very different, but, for introductory teaching purposes, they have enough in common to make comparison valid. When the hydrogen nucleus is placed in a strong magnetic field, it exhibits properties in many ways comparable to those of the compass needle in the earth's magnetic field. It tends to align with the magnetic field; it has a resonant frequency that is proportional to the external field strength; it absorbs energy (provided the energy is at the resonant frequency); and it subsequently re-emits this energy.

In Chapter 2, we learned that a magnetic object (a compass needle) in a magnetic field exhibits magnetic resonance. *When the resonating magnetic object is an atomic nucleus, this is nuclear magnetic resonance (NMR).* The use of NMR to produce images of the body is called *magnetic resonance imaging* (MRI).

Alignment with an External Field

The compass needle has a north pole and a south pole and, in the earth's field, it aligns itself north–south. Similarly, the hydrogen nucleus has a north pole and a south pole and tends to align itself with a strong magnetic field. A fundamental component of an MRI scanner is a means of producing a strong, constant magnetic field.

Resonant Frequency

The frequency at which the hydrogen nucleus oscillates in a magnetic field is its resonant frequency, comparable to the frequency at which the compass needle oscillates in the earth's magnetic field. A term commonly used for the resonant frequency of an atomic nucleus is *Larmor frequency*, named after the British physicist, Sir Joseph Larmor (1857–1942).

A compass needle in the earth's field might oscillate at 1 cycle per second. The resonant (Larmor) frequency of the hydrogen nucleus in the magnetic field of the MRI scanner is many millions of times faster, due both to the physical dimensions and magnetic

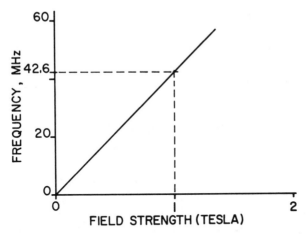

FIG. 3–3. The resonant Larmor frequency of the hydrogen nucleus is directly proportional to field strength.

properties of the hydrogen nucleus and to the much stronger magnetic fields used in MRI. A typical high field strength scanner might have a field strength of 10,000 gauss (one tesla). In this field, the resonant frequency of hydrogen is 42.6 million cycles per second (Figure 3–3).

Stimulation

We were able to stimulate the compass needle into oscillation with a simple tap of our finger, or with a series of light taps. The nucleus of a hydrogen atom is stimulated by another means: radio waves. A radio wave is a weak magnetic field that reverses direction millions of times per second. This alternating field is created by a loop of wire in which the flow of current is constantly reversed at the desired frequency. Each cycle of reversal is the equivalent of a single tap in the series of taps we used to stimulate a compass needle, or of a single push on a child's playground swing.

Radio waves travel at the speed of light and have a particular frequency (the number of cycles per second). For radio waves to be effective in stimulating hydrogen nuclei, the frequency of the radio waves must be tuned to the resonant frequency of the nuclei in a particular magnetic field strength. For the one tesla field mentioned above, the frequency of the radio waves would need to be 42.6 million cycles per second, a frequency located in the short-wave radio band. The radio waves are applied to the hydrogen nuclei in short "bursts" or pulses lasting a small fraction of a second.

Detection of Emitted Energy

The movement of the compass needle could be detected visually, but this is impossible in the case of the hydrogen nucleus. It is nonetheless possible to monitor its behavior because, after stimulation by radio waves of the appropriate frequency, the hydrogen nucleus re-emits the absorbed energy, again in the form of radio waves. These re-emitted waves can be detected by a short-wave radio antenna and receiver.

Another way of explaining this emitted signal is that the nucleus, because it is an oscillating magnet, induces a voltage in an antenna. The signal from an individual nucleus is much too weak to measure, but the signal from many millions of nuclei can be detected by the antenna of the MRI scanner. Quite remarkably, an MRI scanner uses only a short-wave radio transmitter and receiver to stimulate the tissues and to detect the signal from which detailed pictures of the inside of the body are made.

The stimulation of the hydrogen nucleus and detection of its subsequent behavior can be likened to the percussion of a bell: a hammer is used to stimulate the bell, and the energy absorbed from the stimulation is subsequently emitted as sound. A further similarity between sound and NMR is the rate at which the energy is re-emitted. The rate at which the sound of a bell diminishes is comparable to the manner in which hydrogens in tissues re-emit radio energy. In living tissues, this energy falls off over a period of time lasting from perhaps a tenth of a second to a few seconds.

LOCALIZATION OF HYDROGEN NUCLEI

As with the compass needle, the resonant frequency of the stimulated hydrogen nucleus is proportional to the external field strength.

In the case of the compass on the earth's surface, the frequency of its swinging motion increased as we carried it up the magnetic gradient from the Equator toward the North Pole, where the magnetic field is stronger. In MRI, the scanner creates artificial gradients. The gradient field strength changes in a well-defined manner from place to place in the body being scanned. In an MRI scanner's gradient, the location of the hydrogen nucleus can be determined by its resonant frequency.

It is this relationship between magnetic field strength and the resonant frequency of hydrogen nuclei that allows their localization. Localization of hydrogen nuclei in the body is thus similar in principle to localization of a compass needle in the earth's magnetic field. In both cases, location in a gradient field can be deduced from resonant frequency. Without the gradients produced by the MRI scanner, the entire anatomical region under examination would respond as a single entity and no localization within it would be possible. The way in which gradient magnetic fields are used to make clinically useful images is the subject of the next chapter.

4

Imaging

In the first figure of Chapter 1, we described the X-ray CT scan as accomplishing the following imaginary sequence of steps: The head is frozen and a fine saw makes two transverse cuts 1 centimeter apart, thereby creating a cross-sectional slab of head 1 centimeter thick. This slice is removed intact, placed on high-contrast X-ray film and exposed to a broad beam of X-rays at right angles to the slice of tissue. When the radiograph of the slice has been processed and placed on a viewbox, the image would be essentially the same as that produced by the CT scanner. Of course, the CT scanner produces these results without physically altering the head. The slight tissue ionization resulting from this process is entirely harmless (Figure 1–1).

The MRI scan can be described in a similar imaginary fashion. Again, the head is frozen and a transverse slice of tissue cut from it. But after the frozen slice of tissue is removed, rather than a radiograph being made of it, it is physically cut up into tiny square cylinders called *volume elements*, or *voxels*. Each is about one millimeter on an edge and occupies a known position in the original slice of tissue (Figure 4–1). Each of these small square cylinders is, in effect, placed in a test tube that is then placed in a laboratory NMR apparatus, and its hydrogen nuclei are analyzed. This imaginary exercise suggests the great analytic capability of the MRI process. In this chapter, we discuss how MRI localizes these square cylinders of tissue, analyzes them, and then reassembles them to make an image of the cross-sectional slice.

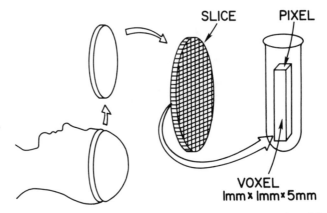

FIG. 4–1. The MRI scan may be thought of as being produced by these steps: freezing the body, cutting out a slab of tissue, slicing it up into small square cylindrical voxels, and placing each voxel in a test tube. The analysis of individual voxels symbolizes the considerable characterization possible by MRI.

NMR IN A UNIFORM FIELD:
ANALYSIS OF A SMALL SAMPLE

We have emphasized the importance of gradient fields in MRI, but, before proceeding to show how gradient fields are used to create an image of a cross-sectional slice, it might be helpful to examine the behavior of a homogeneous sample of hydrogen nuclei in a uniform magnetic field. This will serve to contrast the use of gradient fields with the use of uniform fields, and at the same time give us some idea of what traditional NMR analysis of small samples is like. To carry out the analysis, we could use a simple apparatus similar to that used by Felix Bloch and Robert Purcell, who, independently, described the phenomenon of NMR in 1946.

In this device, a small sample of homogeneous substance (in this case water) is placed in a small test tube, which is placed in the NMR apparatus. The magnetic field applied to the sample is designed to be uniform (1 tesla) throughout the sample. Each hydrogen nucleus in the test tube experiences the same 1 tesla field, and consequently has the same resonant frequency (42.6 million cycles per second) regardless of its location in the test tube. When a stimu-

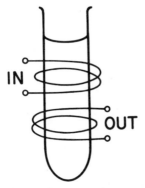

FIG. 4–2. To demonstrate the phenomenon of NMR requires only a simple apparatus. A small test tube filled with a homogeneous sample (water) is placed in a uniform 1 tesla field, and two loops of wire are wrapped around it. One acts as a radio transmitter, exposing the sample to radio energy at the resonant frequency of the hydrogen, and the other as a radio antenna that measures the radio signal re-radiated from the sample. Because the test tube is exposed to a uniform magnetic field, the entire sample responds similarly.

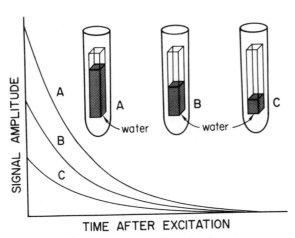

FIG. 4–3. Voxels containing 75%, 50%, and 25% water (respectively) are excited by a radio pulse at the hydrogen resonant frequency. The signal returned from each sample is proportional to the amount of water in the test tube. Measuring regional hydrogen distribution is the simplest MRI analysis.

lating pulse of 42.6 million cycle-per-second radio waves is applied to the sample, the entire sample absorbs the radio-frequency energy. Subsequently, the entire sample re-emits this energy. Because the field within the test tube is uniform, all of the hydrogen nuclei re-emit the energy as 42.6 million cycle-per-second radio waves (Figure 4–2).

An analysis of this re-emitted signal provides information about the hydrogen nuclei. The initial strength of the signal indicates concentration; the observed rate of fading of the signal also tells much about impurities in the water (this will be covered in more detail in the next chapter). But because all of the hydrogen nuclei in the sample respond identically, the signal contains no information that helps to localize hydrogen within the sample (Figure 4–3).

PROPERTIES OF THE HYDROGEN NUCLEUS: A REVIEW

In the previous chapter, we noted the properties of the hydrogen nucleus that are important to MRI:

1. In the presence of the strong magnetic field created in the MRI scanner, the hydrogen nuclei tend to align themselves with the field.

2. The hydrogen nuclei resonate at a frequency (the Larmor frequency) that is proportional to the strength of the magnetic field.

3. In a gradient magnetic field, the resonant frequency of the hydrogen nuclei indicates their physical location.

The MRI scanner creates both the strong field necessary to align the hydrogen nuclei and the gradient fields necessary to localize them. The scanner has a radio transmitter to provide the stimulation (the pulse of radio waves) and an antenna to measure the radio waves re-emitted from the hydrogen nuclei following stimulation.

IMAGING A CROSS-SECTION OF TISSUE

The following section explains how, in a gradient magnetic field, the properties of hydrogen nuclei are used to image a transverse slice of tissue. (Although a transverse slice is used as an example, it is possible to image planes in any orientation.) What follows is a description of the most common method of MRI excitation and data manipulation. Many modifications of this basic method have been described, but the principles are the same.

The first step in imaging a transverse slice is isolation of that slice from other slices. This corresponds to the first step in the imaginary analogy described above: the sawing of the slice of tissue from the body. The most common method of imaging uses gradients to selectively excite an individual slice. After excitation, further information is obtained by creating new gradients within the slice itself. Finally, computer analysis creates the MRI image.

Isolation of a Transverse Slice of Tissue

To isolate this slice, the scanner creates a magnetic gradient longitudinally through the body, from head to foot. (Using X, Y, and Z coordinates, this is termed the *Z-axis*.) We will arbitrarily say that the field is stronger toward the head and weaker toward the feet. In practice, the magnetic gradients used in MRI are weak, changing strength by about 1 gauss per centimeter, which in a 1 tesla field is a change of only 0.01% per centimeter. But the resonance of the hydrogen nucleus is so sharply defined that even such a slight change in field strength is sufficient to isolate a plane a few millimeters thick. It is impractical to create a precisely controlled gradient throughout the entire length of the body, so the gradient is generated only in the region being imaged.

In the presence of this gradient, the hydrogens in the body become spatially encoded, i.e., there is a relationship between their resonant frequency and their position in the gradient. In this example, the hydrogen nuclei in each successively rostral (toward the head) transverse plane of the body are exposed to progressively higher field strengths and so resonate at correspondingly higher Larmor frequencies. As shown in Figure 4–4, there is only one plane of tissue exposed to a field strength of exactly 1 tesla (Figure 4–4). If the entire anatomical region under examination (in this case the head) is exposed to a radio signal of 42.6 million cycles per second, only those hydrogen nuclei lying within the 1 tesla plane of tissue

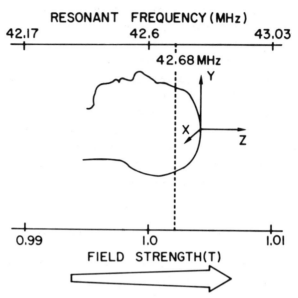

FIG. 4–4. The head is placed in a longitudinal gradient, which is weaker on the left and stronger on the right. The resonant frequencies of hydrogen nuclei vary according to their position in the gradient; a single resonant frequency corresponds to a single transverse plane. When the entire head is exposed to a radio signal of 42.68 megahertz, only the hydrogens in a single transverse slice of tissue (*dashed line*) are stimulated.

absorb the energy of the radio waves and are stimulated. Hydrogen nuclei in adjacent slices of tissue remain unstimulated and "silent." If we wished to isolate a slice of tissue higher or lower in the body, we would adjust the frequency of the radio signal to a higher or lower frequency; we could also change the gradient in relation to the body.

In this way, through the application of a gradient to the body, and the exposure of the tissue to a radio signal of a single frequency, the hydrogen nuclei in only one transverse slice are stimulated. The plane is thus isolated from neighboring, unstimulated tissue. The slice of tissue so isolated can thus be described, using X, Y, and Z coordinates: if the Z-axis is longitudinal through the body, the slice of tissue lies in the X-Y plane.

In this theoretical discussion, we have used a stimulating pulse of radio signal containing only a single frequency. This would produce an infinitesimally thin slice of tissue, and thus an unusable, weak re-emitted signal. In practice, the stimulating pulse would also contain radio frequencies slightly above and below the frequency at the center of the slice. This increases the thickness of the imaged section and increases its signal output.

Localization within the Transverse Slice

At this point we have isolated a slice of tissue by stimulating the hydrogens in only one plane of the body. The hydrogen nuclei start to re-emit the signal immediately after stimulation. But simply stopping the imaging process at this stage and listening to the signal would not provide useful imaging data. All the nuclei in the plane have the same resonant frequency and so emit a radio signal of the same frequency. The intensity of the signal would simply indicate the average signal from all regions of the slice. To further localize the nuclei within the excited slice, new gradients (in different directions) are used.

After the transverse slice of tissue has been isolated and the hydrogens in it stimulated, both the head-to-toe Z-axis gradient and the radio-frequency excitation are turned off. The re-radiated signal appears. A second gradient is then created, this time transversely across the body (at right angles to the Z-axis) in the X-Y plane. As a result, the field on one edge of the slice being imaged is stronger than on the other. How the scanner creates this second gradient will be discussed in Chapter 7. Here, it is important to know only that the transverse gradient can be in any direction across the isolated slice. For simplicity, in Figure 4–5, it is shown increasing from left to right along the X-axis, from ear to ear (Figure 4–5).

The result of applying the second (transverse) gradient is that the nuclei in the isolated slice of tissue, which had all been resonating at the same frequency, now find themselves in magnetic fields of varying strengths. The nuclei resonate at new frequencies, which are higher or lower depending on their positions in the transverse gradient at that instant of time. Again the resonant frequencies of the nuclei are spatially encoded, so that nuclei at one edge of the slice, in the weaker end of the gradient field, resonate at lower frequencies

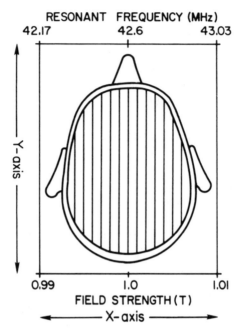

RESONANT FREQUENCY (MHz)

FIG. 4–5. The isolated plane of tissue is exposed to a transverse gradient. Field strength along the X-axis gradient is shown at bottom, and the corresponding hydrogen frequencies at the top. Nuclei along one line have the same resonant frequency.

than those at the other edge, in the stronger field. Thus the excited transverse section of tissue is "sliced" into parallel strips, the nuclei along any one strip resonating at the same frequency (Figure 4–5). A comparable spatial encoding of position by frequency is found in the ordinary piano, in which keys on the left correspond to lower notes and keys on the right to higher. The location of a string on the piano can be determined from the frequency (pitch) of the note produced by the string after being struck (Figure 4–6).

The second magnetic gradient is applied immediately after the original Z-axis gradient is turned off, while the hydrogen nuclei are still "ringing" from their initial stimulation. When they take up their new resonant frequencies in the second gradient, they continue to emit radio-frequency signals without further stimulation. The fre-

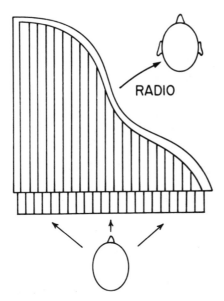

FIG. 4–6. A piano is an example of spatial encoding by frequency. To the left of the keyboard the notes are lower, to the right, higher. Even over the radio, we can determine the location of the strings from their pitch.

quencies of the signals emitted, however, change to correspond to those of the new field strength of the gradient at each left-to-right location, each frequency representing one line across the slice. Regardless of the initial frequency of stimulation, subsequent frequency of oscillation of the nucleus changes with the field strength. This can be compared to the tuning of a guitar string whose pitch instantaneously changes as the tension on the string is adjusted (Figure 4–7).

The radio signal emitted from the plane now contains a mix of frequencies. By measuring the strength of the radio signal at the different frequencies, the amount of hydrogen along each line in the slice of tissue can be determined. This plane of tissue, divided into parallel lines (each line of tissue radiating a specific frequency of radio waves at a particular intensity), can again be compared to a piano. In this case, all of the strings of the piano are vibrating, each

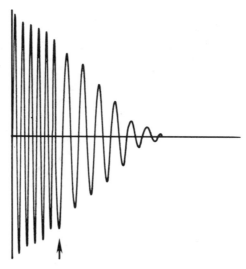

FIG. 4–7. The sound from a guitar string being tuned. The guitar string is plucked and initially oscillates (vibrates) at a specific frequency. The tension on the string is subsequently lowered (*small vertical arrow*). Its frequency of oscillation slows; the pitch of the note drops.

producing its own note. Such a mix of notes would be a meaningless jumble of sound, even to a skilled musician. With the help of electronic frequency analyzers, however, this cacophony could be analyzed into intelligible information. The individual notes could be distinguished, and their respective loudness measured. We would know which notes were being played and how loud they were being played. From this we would know the location of the strings and how hard the corresponding keys had been struck (Figure 4–8).

In MRI such electronic frequency analyzers are used to analyze the radio signal radiating from the tissue. This analysis determines which frequencies are being radiated from the tissues, and at what intensities. The frequency tells us the location of the line; the amplitude tells us the total number of hydrogen nuclei along that line.

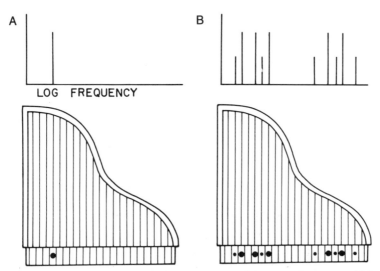

FIG. 4–8. A: Electronic analysis of the sound from a piano on which a single key has been struck (indicated by the black dot on the keyboard). A single peak shows on the electronic display. **B:** Frequency analysis of the sound from a piano on which many keys have been struck with differing intensities (indicated by size of black dot on keyboard). Electronic analysis shows a peak for each key struck. Height of peak indicates how hard the key was struck.

Rotation of the Transverse Gradient

To create an image of a plane of tissue, measurements must be made of many lines criss-crossing the plane. The above describes how data from only one set of parallel lines have been measured. In this section, we describe how data from other lines within the plane are also measured.

After the data retrieved from one pulse have all been recovered and stored in the computer, the excitation and retrieval process described above is repeated, starting with the restoration of the Z-axis gradient. The same transverse slice of tissue across the head is again excited by radio frequency energy. After the stimulating pulse, the Z-axis gradient is again turned off, and the transverse gradient is applied across the isolated slice of tissue, but this time in a slightly

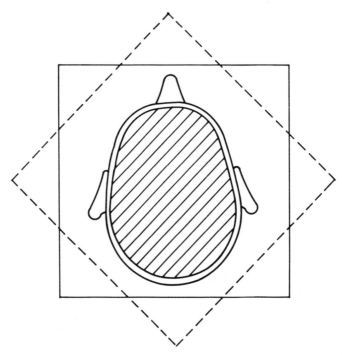

FIG. 4–9. In order to gather enough data to form an image, a single slice of tissue must be examined many times, each time using a transverse gradient oriented in a different direction. Each change of direction defines the number of hydrogens along a new set of parallel lines. Two gradient directions are indicated here (*solid and dashed lines*).

different direction. In this way the hydrogen concentration along a new set of parallel strips, slightly at an angle to the first set, is measured (Figure 4–9). In the course of scanning one slice of tissue, this process is repeated many times. Each time, the transverse gradient is applied to the slice of tissue at a slightly different angle, so that, by the end of the scan, the slice of tissue has been "cut up" into a few hundred sets of parallel lines, each set crossing the plane of the slice at a different angle.

Computer Reconstruction

At this point, we have isolated the slice of tissue from the body and cut it into parallel strips, but we have yet to divide each strip into individual volumes of tissue (voxels) and to measure their hydrogen concentration, as we had proposed. This last step in the imaging process is accomplished by computer.

When the instrumentation in the MRI scanner measures the total amount of hydrogen along a particular strip of tissue in the slice being imaged, the measurement is stored in a computer. Graphically, we can think of this strip as a line having a shade of gray, or *brightness*, that depends on the total amount of hydrogen in the corresponding strip of tissue. During the imaging of one slice of tissue, thousands of such lines of varying brightness are stored in the computer. Any one voxel in the tissue slice represents the intersection of hundreds of lines (Figure 4–10). One might think that the simple superimposition of these lines would result in a useable picture. It would be reasonable to assume that, if any one voxel in the plane is high in hydrogen concentration, all the lines passing

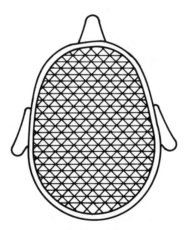

FIG. 4–10. During the course of an MRI scan, the transverse gradient is rotated many times, by a few degrees at a time. The image is reconstructed from the thousands of intersecting lines.

through it would be correspondingly bright and that superimposing these lines should produce a correspondingly bright *picture element*, or *pixel*, and consequently a useable picture. But this is not the case: Such simple superimposition, without further manipulation by computation, results in a blurred and useless picture.

To produce a useable picture, the computer carries out a classical mathematical maneuver—the fourier transform—to reconstruct a clinically useful picture from the data. This involves essentially the same set of instructions (algorithm) used in reconstructing a CT image. The details of the fourier transform and its applications to computer reconstruction of medical images is beyond the scope of this work. (See Oldendorf 1980.)

COMPARISON OF MRI AND CT
COMPUTER RECONSTRUCTION

It is important to point out that the similarities between the computer reconstruction in CT and MRI arise from similarities in the data: Both modalities provide a means for isolating a slice of tissue from the body; both techniques measure some average characteristic along each of a large number of intersecting lines within a plane. In CT, the slice of tissue is isolated by a narrow beam of X-rays, the thickness of the slice of tissue being determined by the width of the X-ray beam. In MRI, the slice of tissue is isolated by radio waves used in combination with a magnetic gradient: hydrogen nuclei in only one slice of tissue respond to stimulation. The thickness of the slice is determined by the range of frequencies used in the exciting radio signal.

CT measures the total density of tissues in a narrow column of tissue interposed between the X-ray source and detector by measuring the fraction of the X-rays lost from the beam as it passes through the head. By changing the position of the source and the detector, the direction and location of the beam are changed.

How the CT scanner measures many lines within a plane of tissue is easiest to understand in the the older (first generation) models of CT scanners. This design used a single X-ray source and detector positioned in the gantry on opposite sides of the patient's head. During the scan, the source and detector were simultaneously moved in parallel motion so that the X-ray beam defined successive, adjacent columns of tissue. In this way, measurements were made of many parallel columns of tissue in the plane being imaged. This parallel movement of the source and detector is termed *translation* (Figure 4–11).

After completing one translation movement across the head, the orientation of the X-ray source and detector was changed so that the direction of the next translational movement was at a different angle

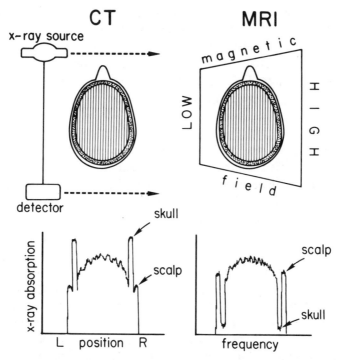

FIG. 4–11. Because CT and MRI both take measurements along many lines crossing a plane of tissue, both use essentially the same computer algorithm to reconstruct an image. MRI measures the number of hydrogen nuclei along each line of tissue; CT measures X-ray absorption between source and detector. One major difference between CT and MRI is shown by the lower profiles: whereas bone in skull strongly absorbs X-rays (and appears bright on CT scans), no radio signal is emitted by bone in MRI (so skull is comparatively black).

across the head. (Adjusting the angle at which the apparatus would scan the head is termed *rotation*.) Thus, the next set of measurements was of a new set of parallel columns of tissues, slightly at an angle to the previous set. The measurements were all stored in the computer and, as in MRI, were represented graphically as a set of parallel lines of varying shades of gray. The *rotate-translate* process was repeated many times, until a data set of several thousand lines was built up. Each line had a position, direction, and brightness, the latter representing the total number of X-ray deletions along the corresponding line through the patient, but providing no information about the desired structural detail.

In a similar fashion, in MRI, measurements are made of a set of parallel lines in the plane of tissue being imaged; the orientation of this set of lines is defined by the direction of the transverse gradient across the slice. During an MRI scan, the direction of the transverse magnetic gradient is changed many times, a few degrees each time, in a step-wise fashion. In this way, measurements are made of hydrogen nuclei along many intersecting lines through the plane under examination. Again, the exact location of each hydrogen cannot be determined, but their total concentration along each line is measured. The same computerized reconstruction as in X-ray CT is then applied to produce a two-dimensional MRI image, which superficially resembles a CT scan. In the case of MRI, however, the images represent the distribution of hydrogen. (As we will see in Chapter 5, the MRI data-gathering strategy may be modified to display other tissue characteristics [Figure 4–11]).

In the case of CT, changes in direction of successive sweeps through tissue can be made only by mechanically moving the X-ray source. This greatly complicates design, construction, and maintenance of the CT scanner, and confines CT to imaging in the transverse plane. The change in direction of the magnetic field gradients in MRI scanning, however, does not require any physical movement because it can be accomplished electronically, using no moving parts. One result of this is that MRI, unlike CT, is not confined to transverse slices; it can also image coronal or sagittal slices (and any other orientation), since the gradients can be used to create any examination plane desired. Although in this chapter the imaging of a transverse slice of tissue was used as an example, in MRI it is no more difficult to image other planes. To do this, the gradients are applied in different orientations. For example, instead of the first gradient being applied longitudinally along the body, it can be applied transversely across the body to produce a sagittal section, or front-to-back for a coronal section.

SUMMARY

The use of linear gradients to localize an NMR signal was described by Lauterbur (1973), and the success of this early method opened the door to a variety of embellishments of his fundamental approach. The material in this chapter describes essentially Lauterbur's original work and is intended to introduce the principles of MRI.

In this chapter, an image of hydrogen distribution was achieved by exposing the tissues to a single excitation pulse and then measuring the signal re-emitted from the tissues. In fact, a single excitation pulse is rarely used in modern imaging. As described in Chapter 5, two or more pulses are usually used to emphasize other characteristics of the hydrogen nucleus and so better characterize tissues.

5

Tissue Characterization

Up to this point, we have discussed only one capability of MRI: the mapping of hydrogen concentration. If this were the only capability of MRI, it probably would not be worth the major effort already undertaken to develop clinical scanners. The great potential of MRI derives from its ability to provide several means of characterizing normal and pathological tissues.

We ordinarily think of tissue analysis as the measurement of the amount of a given substance per unit volume of tissue, for example, the amount of glucose in a volume of serum. In CT, measurements are made of regional specific gravity and iodine concentration. The simplest method of MRI scanning shows regional concentration of hydrogen nuclei, because the signal strength immediately after a single pulse is proportional to the number of hydrogen nuclei. Most hydrogens are in tissue water and fat. In practice, such simple hydrogen imaging turns out to be of little interest because there is so much hydrogen in essentially all tissues that there is little regional contrast. The useful information lies almost entirely in the *behavior* of regional hydrogen, rather than in its regional concentration. Here, what is meant by behavior is how the hydrogen nucleus responds to influences from its chemical environment. The chemical environment changes the behavior of the hydrogen nucleus, which in turn changes the qualities of the NMR radio signal emitted by the tissues.

The idea of using the hydrogen nucleus to tell us about its environment may be clarified by a simple analogy. Through experience, we have learned how people respond to changes in the weather. Imagine that you awaken in a hotel room in a strange city and wish to know what the weather is like outside. If you looked out the window and could see people on the street below, you could infer much about the weather by observing their behavior. They serve as a behavioral probe of the weather. How are they dressed? If they are without coats it is probably warm. If they have umbrellas opened, it is most likely raining. If they are rushing about, it has probably just begun to rain. If they seek shelter in protected areas, it may be windy. There are many other inferences about the weather that could be drawn from human behavior. Simply counting the people would be only a crude indicator of the weather.

In MRI we observe the hydrogen nucleus and infer characteristics of its magnetic environment from its behavior. By varying the nature of the radio-frequency probe, we can elicit different types of information. During the short period of time following stimulation, the behavior of hydrogen nuclei becomes a surprisingly rich source of information about the magnetic "weather" in the tissues.

CHANGES IN BEHAVIOR DUE TO
LOCAL MAGNETIC FIELDS

To show how the behavior of hydrogen nuclei allows us to infer their environment, we might return briefly to the compass analogy. We must first emphasize that the compass is only a crude approximation of the properties of the hydrogen nucleus. A large number of compass needles behave collectively like a large number of hydrogen nuclei; but while a single compass needle is used to make a point, it is not closely representative of the processes involved with a single hydrogen nucleus.

At different parallels of latitude, the compass needle swings or oscillates at different resonant frequencies, because field strength varies according to distance from the poles. If we carry the compass needle to different locations at the same latitude, we would expect it to oscillate at exactly the same frequency, since any point at that latitude is equidistant from the pole and should experience the same strength magnetic field. In fact, we would find that the resonant frequency of the compass varies slightly with even minor changes of location. These changes are due to small local variations in the strength of the earth's field. At one location, the compass might be near a natural deposit of iron ore, at another it might be inside a building with steel beams. These factors would change the strength of the magnetic field experienced by the compass needle.

RELAXATION TIMES

The hydrogen nucleus exposed to the magnetic field created by the MRI scanner likewise experiences small local variations in magnetic field strength. These fluctuations occur on a submolecular level, due to the presence of magnetic nuclei and atoms. Hydrogen nuclei are themselves weakly magnetic; but there are also other atoms and molecules in tissues, such as manganese and dissolved oxygen, that are very strongly magnetic. The nuclear magnetism of water hydrogen and other atoms is not obvious, since it is not apparent in ordinary physiology, but these magnetic nuclei and magnetic atoms significantly alter the magnetic microenvironment of the water hydrogens being imaged. These effects are the "weather" in our earlier hotel window analogy. It is the ability to detect these differences in the magnetic environment of the hydrogen nucleus that gives MRI its great diagnostic potential.

These alterations in behavior modify the signal emitted by the hydrogen nuclei after excitation. There are two observable aspects of behavior of the hydrogen nucleus that are affected by the local magnetic environment: these are termed *time constants* T_1 and T_2. They are also referred to as *relaxation times* since they define the rate at which emitted signal fades (relaxes) after stimulation. T_1 and T_2 represent two quite independent processes, each of which contributes to fading of the signal following excitation.

Time Constant T_1 (Compass Needle)

To understand T_1, we can examine the behavior of one compass needle on the earth's surface. First we stimulate the compass needle by tapping it with our finger. Initially, it swings in a wide arc as it oscillates. Over a period of several seconds, the needle loses kinetic energy to bearing friction and air drag, swinging in progressively shorter arcs until it finally comes to rest, pointing north. The com-

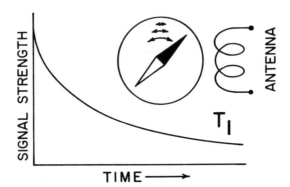

FIG. 5–1. The swinging compass needle loses energy due to friction and air drag, eventually returning to rest in its original position in the earth's field. An external antenna measures T_1, the rate of decay.

pass needle, being a small magnet, induces a faint but detectable signal in an antenna coil placed near it. The signal diminishes as the swinging motion diminishes. For mathematical reasons, we define T_1 as the time it takes for the compass needle to lose 63% of its original energy (Figure 5–1).

Time Constant T_2 (Compass Needle)

Imagine that we have several identical compasses, located at different points on the same parallel of latitude on the earth's surface. We stimulate them simultaneously so that they swing in unison. We would expect the motion of the compass needles to decay at the same rate and their observed signals to fall off at the same rate as a single compass. But this is not the case. The combined signal falls off much faster than expected, due to the phenomenon of dephasing. Although the compass needles would all initially be swinging together (in phase), unavoidable local variations in magnetic field strength cause them to swing at slightly different rates; after a few seconds they are no longer in phase. Even though each compass is still swinging, the signal produced by any one compass needle partially cancels that produced by another. Consequently, over a period of a few seconds, the combined observed signal falls off more quickly than the signal from a single compass. T_2, then, is defined

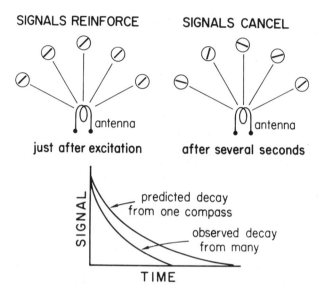

FIG. 5–2. Initially a group of compass needles swing in phase with each other, but local variations in magnetic field strength cause them to oscillate at slightly differing rates. As they drift out of phase, their combined signal falls off at rate T_2.

as the time it takes for dephasing to weaken the signal by 63%. The measured signal can disappear due to dephasing, even though individually the compasses have not lost their energy (Figure 5–2).

It is easy to find examples of mutual reinforcement of multiple weak signals. A platoon of soldiers might be walking along a road some distance from an observer. The sound of their boots on the road might not be audible if they were simply walking out of step with each other. If, however, they were marching in step, the thumping sounds of their individual boots would reinforce each other and be audible at a distance. To say they are marching "in step" is a way of stating they are marching in phase, or that they are phase coherent.

Loss of Energy

T_1 measures the rate of loss of energy; it is important to note that the compass actually loses energy as the oscillation decays, and the needle comes back to rest pointing north. In T_2, there is no energy loss; the weakening of the emitted signal occurs as a group effect, the result of dephasing (a loss of coherence) between the compasses. They are still swinging individually, but their combined signal fades.

T_1 AND T_2 IN MRI

In the watery environment of the body's tissues, hydrogen nuclei (in the aggregate) also exhibit these two properties. When the human body is exposed to the brief stimulating pulse from the MRI scanner's radio transmitter, many trillions of nuclei are stimulated in the slice of tissue being imaged. Immediately, two processes start: the re-emission of energy, measured as T_1, and the dephasing of oscillating hydrogen nuclei, measured as T_2. The radio signal re-emitted from the tissues is measured by the MRI scanner's antenna and radio receiver; the decay of the observed signal occurs due to the combined effects of T_1 and T_2. Fortunately, it is possible to measure the individual contributions of T_1 and T_2 to signal fading.

T_1 of Hydrogen

T_1 is defined as the time it takes for the hydrogen nuclei to emit 63% of the energy they absorbed from the stimulating pulse. At field strengths ordinarily used in MRI scanners, the T_1 of pure water is about 2.5–3 seconds.

T_2 of Hydrogen

One effect of the stimulating radio frequency pulse is to make all of the hydrogen nuclei oscillate more or less in phase with each other, just as tapping a group of compass needles simultaneously made them swing in phase. Immediately after the excitation, they are maximally in phase. As they continue to oscillate, the movement of magnetic nuclei and atoms creates minute, fluctuating local magnetic fields. These cause the hydrogen nuclei to oscillate at slightly different frequencies, causing them to drift out of phase with each other. Eventually they become completely out of phase. When the nuclei oscillate out of phase, the radio waves they emit are also out of phase and so act to cancel each other. As a result, the signal detected by the MRI scanner—the sum of radio signals from trillions of nuclei—falls off more quickly than if the nuclei were unaffected by local fluctuations. T_2 is defined as the time for 63% of the signal to be lost due to dephasing. T_2 of pure water is comparable to T_1, about 2.5–3 seconds.

(We should note that T_2 must always be shorter than or equal to T_1, since phase relationship is of no interest once the nuclei have all lost their energy.)

FACTORS AFFECTING T_1 AND T_2

To some extent it is possible to isolate a compass needle from extraneous magnetic influences so that it responds only to the earth's magnetic field. In the watery environment of the tissues, it is impossible to isolate a hydrogen nucleus from local magnetic influences so that it responds only to the field of the MRI scanner. Water molecules are in constant motion, dynamically interacting with other magnetic nuclei and atoms, which can have a strong influence on the measured magnetic properties of the hydrogen nuclei. The most we can do to reduce extraneous magnetic influences is to remove magnetic impurities from the water, but, even in pure water, the magnetic hydrogen nuclei influence each other.

In pure water, T_1 and T_2 of hydrogen have approximately the same value—about 2.5 seconds. In living tissues, the complex microenvironments strongly influence the magnetic properties of water molecules: both T_1 and T_2 are greatly shortened, and the signal fades correspondingly faster. The exceptions to this are cerebrospinal fluid and urine, which both behave magnetically much like pure water.

Because T_1 and T_2 are strongly influenced by tissue microenvironments, they provide means of characterizing tissues. To understand tissue characterization in MRI, therefore, it is important to know something about the source of the local magnetic field fluctuations that alter magnetic behavior of hydrogen nuclei.

Thermal Motion

The environment of the nucleus is a world of violent motion. At body temperature, water and other molecules that make up the magnetic environment are in constant motion, colliding randomly with each other.

The most obvious manifestation of this thermal motion is Brownian motion, which was first observed by Scottish botanist Robert Brown in 1827, while examining a suspension of pollen grains under a high power microscope. A pollen grain or other small particle undergoes visible random movement as though buffeted by invisible particles. In the vicinity of the particle are many very much smaller water molecules, bombarding its surface millions of times per second. These impacts on the particle largely cancel each other, but since they are random in time they sometimes impact unequally on two sides of the particle. The result is a jiggling motion of the particle that is low enough in frequency and has enough displacement to be visible with any good microscope. Anyone interested in MRI should seek out an ordinary laboratory microscope and observe India ink (diluted one drop to a cup of water) at 400–1000 magnification. The vigorous motion of the carbon particles that make the ink black is very impressive. It is a direct observation of thermal motion, the basis of both T_1 and T_2 relaxation.

Brownian motion gives the impression that the particles suspended in the water are alive and moving spontaneously. Brown made his original observations using pollen grains that he thought were male. Consequently, he believed their motion was comparable to that of spermatozoa. But he also observed the same motion in what he thought were female pollen grains; he soon established that completely lifeless mineral particles of this size also showed the same motion. Brownian motion, despite its apparent vigor, persists forever, provided the liquid is not allowed to cool below its freezing point. If the liquid freezes, all visible motion ceases. No satisfactory explanation for Brownian motion appeared until 1905 when, in one of his four classic papers of that year, Albert Einstein mathematically analyzed the process of diffusion. Unaware that Brownian motion had been observed decades earlier, Einstein predicted that it should be seen if looked for.

Water molecules undergo similar random collisions with each other but, being very much smaller than India ink particles, they undergo collisions at a much faster rate (Figure 5–3). It is important to note that, in addition to direct collisions, many near collisions also occur. Since water molecules contain two magnetic hydrogen nuclei, each interaction of one water molecule with another— whether a collision or near collison—is a magnetic event resulting in a brief fluctuation of the magnetic field experienced by each nucleus. Because a water molecule undergoes millions of collisions per second, each nucleus experiences millions of magnetic fluctuations. The hydrogen nuclei in the tissues respond to this magnetic signal, as they did to the electromagnetic radio waves from the MRI scanner's radio transmitter during stimulation.

Whereas the signal produced by a radio transmitter is well controlled, consisting of cycles of fluctuation of the same intensity at evenly spaced intervals, the nature of the magnetic signal produced by thermal motion is much more complex. The collisions or near misses between water molecules occur randomly, so the fluctuations in the local field strength are random. How close the water molecules come to each other in near collisions is also variable, so the intensity of the fluctuations is correspondingly variable. In addi-

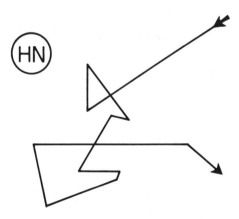

FIG. 5–3. In the liquid state a water molecule moves rapidly, changing direction and rotating as it undergoes many collisions and near collisions.

tion, other aspects of the molecule's motion create magnetic perturbations. First, each collision changes the speed, as well as the direction, of the water molecule. Second, the molecule undergoes a
rotational tumbling motion as it moves. These additional motions of
the water molecules further complicate the magnetic fluctuations, or
signal, experienced by other water molecules. Consequently, the
magnetic field produced within a region of water by thermal motion
is extremely complex. It can be thought of as a mixture of magnetic
fluctuations covering a wide range of frequencies.

The complexity of these randomly produced magnetic influences
can be compared to the familiar phenomenon of audible *white noise*.
When an inflated tire is punctured, we hear a hiss as the air escapes
into the atmosphere. The hissing is the result of the turbulence created when the rapid stream of air emerges from the hole, is broken
into many vortices, and mixes with the surrounding still air. This
turbulence is a random phenomenon that produces a wide range of
audible frequencies, called *white noise*. The term *white noise* is bor-
rowed from the field of optics, which tells us that the color white is
produced by a mixture of all frequencies (colors) of visible light. In
tissues, the complex thermal motion of water molecules produces a
comparable phenomenon, a magnetic signal containing fluctuations
occurring at many frequencies. This is the environment of magnetic
white noise to which the hydrogen nucleus responds during the MRI
imaging process. The responses of hydrogen nuclei to environmental magnetic fluctuations determine the rate of energy loss (T_1) and
the rate of dephasing (T_2) during MRI.

Effect of Thermal Motion on T_2

(Because the effect of thermal motion on the T_2 of hydrogen is
more easily explained than for T_1, it is presented here first.)

We have seen how the resonant Larmor frequency of the hydrogen nucleus depends upon the strength of the magnetic field it experiences. In MRI scanning, almost all of this field is produced by the
scanner itself. But thermal motion of tissue water is constantly creating minute fluctuations that are superimposed on this main field.
Any fluctuation results in a corresponding change in the resonant
frequency and causes the nucleus to oscillate slightly faster or

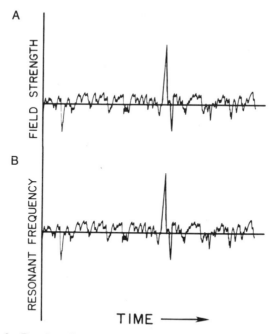

FIG. 5–4. A. Random fluctuations in field strength at a particular nucleus, due to the thermal motion of magnetic nuclei and atoms. In this imaginary graph, the large spike represents a very near miss with a strongly magnetic atom. **B.** The resonant frequency of the nucleus varies, precisely following changes in field strength. The random change in resonant frequency of each nucleus causes the degradation of phase relationship between nuclei, thereby determining T_2.

slower. Since no two nuclei experience the same fluctuations, the oscillations of the nuclei, over a period of time, drift out of phase with each other (Figure 5–4).

During MRI, large populations of hydrogen nuclei are stimulated by a pulse of radio-frequency energy; subsequently, they re-emit the energy, again as radio waves. The strength of the received signal does not represent the amount of energy being re-emitted; the emitted energy seems to disappear long before it actually does because the nuclear sources creating the signal go rapidly out of phase.

To summarize T_2 (the loss of signal due to dephasing): Immediately after stimulation the Larmor precessions of the nuclei are most in phase. At this time, the emitted radio waves (which, when summed, create the observed signal) are in phase, and the signal is strongest. Because the nuclei drift out of phase due to thermal motion, the emitted radio waves drift out of phase and cancel each other, so the radio signal falls off quickly. When they are completely out of phase (randomly phased), no signal is received. As stated above, the rate of dephasing is defined as T_2, the time it takes for the dephasing to cause the signal to fall by 63%. It is important to note that T_2 is shortened by an increase in magnetic noise fluctuations of *any* frequency.

Effect of Thermal Motion on T_1

Hydrogen nuclei being imaged by MRI are stimulated by radio waves tuned to the resonant Larmor frequency of the nuclei. (In a 1 tesla field, the Larmor frequency of hydrogen nuclei is 42.6 million cycles per second.)

In the tissue environment, a very small component of the magnetic white noise caused by thermal motion occurs at the Larmor frequency, the frequency at which the hydrogen nucleus is oscillating. We might expect that magnetic fluctuations at the resonant frequency of the nuclei would evoke a special response from the energized nuclei, and this is indeed the case. For reasons explained in the Appendix on quantum processes, magnetic fluctuations at this particular frequency cause the population of stimulated hydrogen nuclei to lose their energy faster than in the absence of these fluctuations. The magnetic signal triggers the release of energy. This type of event is known as a *stimulated emission*.

To summarize T_1: Immediately after stimulation, the hydrogen nuclei in a sample of tissue contain the most energy. Immediately, they begin to re-emit this energy in the form of radio waves. The magnetic fluctuations produced by thermal motion in the tissue influence the rate at which energy is emitted: the more fluctuations that occur at the Larmor frequency of the nuclei, the faster the energy is emitted. As previously stated, T_1 is defined as the time it takes for thermal noise to make the hydrogen nuclei lose 63% of their energy. While T_2 is affected by magnetic noise fluctuations at *any* frequency, T_1 is affected *only* by those fluctuations at the resonant Larmor frequency.

Effect of Temperature on Thermal Motion, T_1, and T_2

In commercial MRI scanners, the resonant Larmor frequency of hydrogen nuclei falls somewhere in the range of 1–85 million cycles per second, the specific frequency being determined by the strength of the main magnet. In pure water, the thermal motion of water molecules produces a wide range of frequencies, starting at zero cycles per second and extending up into the thousands of millions of cycles per second, far above the Larmor frequencies likely to be found in imaging. In fact, most of the magnetic fluctuations occur at frequencies above the range of the Larmor frequencies found in MRI. Only a small fraction of the magnetic fluctuations produced by thermal noise occurs at the lower Larmor frequencies. Of these, only a very small fraction occurs at the specific Larmor frequency of a particular MRI scanner. This small component at the Larmor frequency does have an important effect, however, triggering the hydrogen nuclei being imaged to lose their energy. The strength of this particular frequency component thus determines T_1.

Temperature has a direct effect on thermal motion and, consequently, on the magnetic noise and T_1. At body temperature, thermal motion of pure water tends to be "high-pitched," most of its magnetic noise occurring above the range of MRI Larmor frequencies. When water is cooled, thermal motion slows. The magnetic fluctuations shift down into a lower frequency range, and more occur at MRI Larmor frequencies. More stimulated emissions occur and T_1 shortens. The same effect occurs when the viscosity of water is increased by dissolving large molecules in it: thermal motion slows, and T_1 shortens (Figure 5–5). (While T_1 shortens with decreasing temperature, T_2 does not because it is determined by fluctuations of *any* frequency.)

This shifting of frequencies in magnetic noise again has a parallel in acoustics. We know from experience that audible hissing can be described as "high" or "low." A small hole in an inflated tire produces a higher pitched hissing sound than a larger hole does. Both types of hissing noise contain a wide range of frequencies, but the

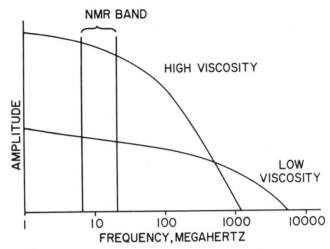

FIG. 5–5. The two curves represent the frequency distribution of the magnetic fluctuations due to thermal motion. At low viscosity (or high temperature), the thermal motion is faster; there are more high-frequency components. The area under the two curves is the same. The hydrogen resonant frequency falls somewhere in the NMR band, depending on the strength of the magnet in the scanner. At high viscosity (or lower temperature), thermal motion slows; more of the fluctuations occur in the NMR band. (Modified from Ferrar and Becker, 1971.)

higher hiss contains more high-pitched frequencies than the lower hiss.

In summary, both T_1 and T_2 measure the responses of hydrogen nuclei to magnetic perturbations from their environment. T_1 is solely a response to a *specific* frequency component in these perturbations—the resonant Larmor frequency of the hydrogen nucleus. T_2 is a response to magnetic perturbations of *any* frequency.

Polar Macromolecules and Microviscosity

Most large molecules of biological interest are polar; they are nearly electrically neutral overall, yet they have an uneven distribution of charge on their surface. These local charge sites attract water molecules, which are also polar. Because of their large size and weight, the thermal movement of macromolecules, such as pro-

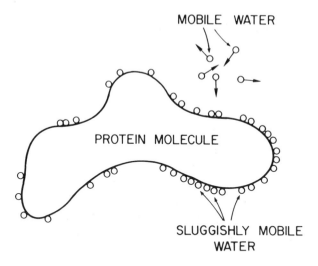

MOBILE WATER

PROTEIN MOLECULE

SLUGGISHLY MOBILE
WATER

MICROVISCOSITY

FIG. 5–6. Due to its large size, a (polar) protein molecule moves much more slowly than freely moving water molecules. Due to its polarity, it attracts the highly polar water molecules to charged sites on its surface, slowing their average motion, and shortening T_1.

teins, is sluggish compared to that of the water in which they are dissolved. Accordingly, the thermal motion of water molecules attached to the surface of the macromolecule, or in its vicinity, is greatly slowed. We could see this effect in an ocean liner and a nearby fleet of dinghies. If a fleet of dinghies is exposed to choppy water, the small boats pitch to and fro in a rapid movement, whereas the motion of the ocean liner remains relatively steady. If we tied the small boats to the ocean liner, their movement would stabilize and be slowed (Figure 5–6).

The effect of polar macromolecules on the thermal motion of water is similar to the effect of cooling the water. In both cases, the motion of the water molecules is slowed, and the frequencies of magnetic fluctuations produced by this motion are lowered. More magnetic fluctuations now occur at the resonant Larmor frequency of the nucleus and, as a result, the rate of stimulated emission and energy loss is accelerated; T_1 of the water is shortened. Whether due to dissolved macromolecules or to cooling, slower thermal motion shortens T_1 of water hydrogen in body tissues, but has no effect on T_2.

Paramagnetism: A Product of Orbiting Electrons

Many atoms exhibit magnetic properties that are due not to the properties of the nucleus, but to the structure of their circulating clouds of electrons.

In Chapter 3, we learned a simple rule of thumb that allowed a prediction of whether a particular nucleus would be magnetic (Figure 3–2). Nuclear magnetism results from the property of nuclear spin possessed by protons and neutrons. The spin of one neutron cancels the spin of its paired neutron, and similarly for protons. When the nucleus possesses an odd number of either protons or neutrons, the spin of the extra unpaired proton or neutron creates the magnetic field of the nucleus. Since the spin of a neutron cannot cancel that of a proton, if the nucleus contains both an unpaired proton and unpaired neutron, the nucleus is still magnetic.

Electrons orbit a nucleus. This roughly circular motion of a charge produces a magnetic field in the same way that electrons moving in a circular wire produce a field. The prediction of the magnetic behavior of these orbiting electrons is complicated by the fact that, like all fundamental particles, electrons possess spin. The spin of each electron on its axis creates its own magnetic field. This magnetic effect is superimposed on that due to orbital motion, so the overall magnetic field of the electron is the sum of these two components. In some atoms, such as the noble gases (helium, neon, argon, etc.), which have no unpaired electrons, the magnetic fields from both the spin and orbital motion of the various electrons completely cancel each other, and the atom is not magnetic. In other atoms, these two factors—orbital motion and spin—do not cancel, and consequently the atom is magnetic. Atoms that are magnetic due to the effects of orbiting electrons are called *paramagnetic* (Figure 5–7).

Because of these two effects, and because of the variable number of electrons of a given element in various valence states, there is no simple rule allowing us to predict whether a given atom will be

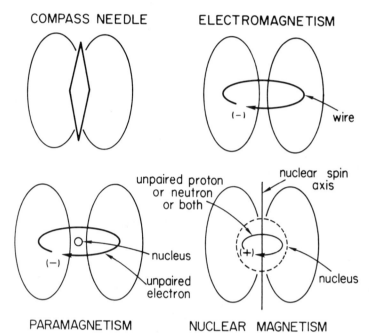

FIG. 5–7. In Chapter 3 we learned that an atomic nucleus is magnetic if it possesses a net spin from unpaired protons or neutrons (see Figures 3–1 and 3–2). Electrons orbiting the nucleus may also produce magnetism due to their orbital motion and spin. This paramagnetism is much stronger than nuclear magnetism.

paramagnetic. (The terms paramagnetism and ferromagnetism are easily confused. Ferromagnetic atoms are paramagnetic atoms that, when placed in a magnetic field, become magnetized by aligning with the external field, and that, to some degree, remain aligned and thus magnetized after the field is removed. Paramagnetic atoms also align with the field but do not retain their alignment after removal of the field.)

Examples of Paramagnetic Atoms and Molecules

Many atoms are paramagnetic to some degree, but there is a great range; the magnetism produced by the stronger paramagnetic atoms is about 1,000 times greater than a hydrogen nucleus. Because nuclear magnetism is trivial in magnitude compared to paramagnetism, it can be studied only because magnetic nuclei are highly resonant at specific frequencies. Their magnetism would otherwise be overshadowed by the much stronger atomic magnetism (paramagnetism) due to electrons.

Some of the transitional elements in the middle of the periodic table show especially strong paramagnetism. Two of these, manganese and gadolinium have been studied extensively in clinical MRI because they are strongly paramagnetic. Gaseous oxygen (O_2) in solution is also strongly paramagnetic, although the reasons for this are obscure and a discussion of this topic would be beyond the scope of this book. Inhaled O_2 has been used successfully as a tracer in MRI, but little long-term interest has been shown. Fortunately, covalently bonded oxygen, such as that in water, is not paramagnetic. (If it were, its strong contribution to thermal noise probably would preclude any nuclear magnetic studies of tissues.)

The outer electron shells of a given element can have different numbers of electrons. These determine the valence of the atom, and thus their chemical reactivity. Usually, when there is an even number of electrons in a given valence state, the atom is not paramagnetic. But an odd number of electrons in either of the outer two shells usually results in an unpaired electron, making the atom paramagnetic. The element gadolinium can have seven unpaired electrons and, accordingly, is strongly paramagnetic. These generalizations concerning the relationship between outer shell structures and paramagnetism are not always applicable.

The appearance of paramagnetism in blood lying stagnant in tissues can be used to crudely estimate how long the blood has been present. Fresh blood contains hemoglobin, in which iron is in the (Fe^{+++}) form; it is not paramagnetic and, on an MRI scan, it is sometimes difficult to differentiate from adjacent brain. After a few days at body temperature, stagnant hemoglobin is oxidized to methemoglobin, in which iron is in the (Fe^{++}) form , which is paramagnetic. The corresponding shortening of relaxation times may then allow MRI to differentiate the hematoma from adjacent brain.

Paramagnetism and MRI

Paramagnetic atoms play an important role in MRI: In solution, they act as small, strong, randomly moving magnets. As thermal motion carries them through the liquid microenvironments, paramagnetic atoms and molecules have powerful effects on T_1 and especially T_2.

In solution, at body temperature, paramagnetic atoms or molecules undergo the random thermal motion of other atoms and molecules. Because each is so strongly magnetic, a very low concentration of paramagnetic atoms or molecules can have a profound effect on the much weaker magnetic nuclei of nearby atoms. Paramagnetic atoms increase the magnetic white noise and intensify the magnetic fluctuations at all frequencies, including the Larmor frequency, thus affecting both T_1 and T_2.

The increase in fluctuations at the Larmor frequency triggers more T_1 decays, thereby shortening T_1. As we have seen (Figure 5–4), random fluctuations occurring at *any* frequency result in dephasing of the hydrogen nuclei. The increased magnetic noise caused by paramagnetic atoms randomly changes the field strength at nearby nuclei, resulting in more rapid dephasing and shortening of T_2. The effects of paramagnetic atoms on T_1 and especially T_2 are measurable even in concentrations in the range of one part per million. With the small amount of paramagnetic material injected as contrast agents, the observed effects of paramagnetism are much greater on T_2.

It is difficult to determine the exact effects of paramagnetic substances naturally present in the complex chemical environment of tissues. Gaseous oxygen (O_2) is present in tissues and contributes, to some undetermined extent, to a shortened T_1 and T_2. Other elements, such as copper and iron, are present in very small concentrations and may also affect T_1 and T_2 in minor ways. Certain nerve cells in the brain contain about 4 times as much iron as average brain. These nerve cells are found in the red nucleus, substantia nigra, globus, and caudate nuclei. Consequently, the T_2 of these cells is much shorter, and they appear visibly darker than surrounding brain on T_2-weighted scans.

MRI Contrast Agents

One of the main reasons for understanding the phenomenon of paramagnetism is to understand the use of contrast agents in MRI. MRI contrast agents are paramagnetic substances that are artificially introduced into the body in order to create more contrast on the MRI scan. Even small amounts of artificially introduced paramagnetic substances (contrast agents) can have visible effects on T_1 and T_2. Manganese and gadolinium are strongly paramagnetic and have been actively studied as injectable contrast agents. These atoms can be inserted into molecules much as radioactive atoms are inserted into molecules for use in radioisotope scans in nuclear medicine. However, the chemical amounts required for MRI are much greater than those needed for radioisotope scans. Accordingly, chemical toxicity of MRI contrast agents is a much greater concern. (In radio-active studies, toxicity can almost always be ignored because the chemical amount of injected substance is vanishingly small.)

The most common paramagnetic contrast agent currently in use for brain is gadolinium, bound (chelated) into an organic molecule. This appears to be chemically inert and non-toxic, being excreted rapidly in the urine. Gaseous oxygen has also shown promise as a contrast agent; animals inhaling 100% (O_2) show a detectable short-ening of relaxation times in heart muscle. Inhaled 100% O_2 has been used successfully as an MRI contrast agent in humans. Although it is a safe, inexpensive, and simple contrast agent, little long-term clinical interest has been shown in it. (See Chapters 9 and 10 for further discussions of MRI and CT contrast agents.)

THE TERMS *LATTICE* AND *SPIN*

The interaction of excited hydrogen nuclei with their surrounding environment is usually discussed using the terms *lattice* and *spin*. To understand these terms we can consider the interaction of a water molecule with other water molecules as falling into one of two cate-gories: interactions between a few relatively nearby nuclei, and in-teractions between large numbers of nuclei more distant from each other. There is no sharp dividing line between those that are *nearby* and those that are *distant*.

There are relatively few molecules undergoing collisions or near collisions with any one water molecule under examination. Conse-quently, the collisions and near misses are relatively few in number, but each of these creates a strong fluctuation in local magnetic field

$$T_2 \qquad\qquad T_1$$

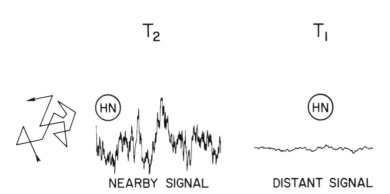

NEARBY SIGNAL   DISTANT SIGNAL

FIG. 5–8. The thermal motion of a magnetic nucleus causes strong random fluctuations in field strength at a nearby hydrogen nucleus (HN), whose Larmor frequency changes proportionately. Because the Larmor frequency of each of the nuclei in a region changes randomly, they become dephased, at a rate described as T_2. At a distant nucleus, such thermal motion produces weak perturbations that have little effect on the Larmor frequency. Perturbations from trillions of other distant sources combine to create a high-frequency magnetic signal containing some component at the resonant larmor frequency, thus triggering T_1 decay.

strength. In a larger volume surrounding the water molecule under examination, there are many more water molecules interacting from a distance. A single water molecule interacting from a distance creates a fluctuation that is relatively weak. The weak fluctuations from these many distant water molecules tend to average out, since they are randomly generated, so distant nuclei rarely create large fluctuations in field strength. Still, the combination of this vast number of feeble magnetic signals contains frequency components ranging from zero to billions of cycles per second (Figure 5–8).

Near Encounters, Distant Encounters:
How They Affect T_1 and T_2

In MRI of hydrogen nuclei, it is the motion of a nearby water molecule or paramagnetic atom that results in large fluctuations of magnetic field strength. Such large fluctuations transiently alter the resonant Larmor frequencies of the nuclei under examination causing them to become dephased from each other. We can see, then, that it is the movement of nearby magnetic particles that produces the strongest effect on T_2. This type of magnetic interaction, which occurs at short range, is called a *spin-spin* interaction. The term *spin* derives from nuclear spin, which is the source of nuclear magnetism. The term *spin* can be interchanged with *magnet*. In *spin-spin* interaction, one magnetic nucleus is interacting directly with relatively few nearby magnetic nuclei or atoms. It could be called a one-on-one, *magnet-magnet* interaction.

The movement of the many distant molecules creates fluctuations in magnetic field strength but, due to distance, the fluctuations are weaker than those created by nearby molecules. Because these fluctuations are weak, and because they are random (and so partially cancel, rather than reinforce, each other) the interactions with distant molecules do not create the intense changes in magnetic field and resonant frequency caused by interaction with nearby water molecules. From this we can see that the interaction with distant molecules has little effect on T_2. The many random, weak fluctuations from distant molecules create a *magnetic noise* containing a wide range of frequencies, extending both above and below likely Larmor frequencies of hydrogen nuclei in MRI scanning. The small fraction of this *lattice noise* occurring at the Larmor frequency has an important effect: it triggers the release of energy from stimulated nuclei, shortening T_1.

The T_1 decay of an excited magnetic nucleus in response to specific magnetic frequency components from the extended environment is traditionally called a *spin-lattice* interaction. The word *spin* again refers to the magnetic nucleus under examination. The term *lattice* refers to the extended environment of the nucleus and tends to de-emphasize the role of individual nearby nuclei in their effect on T_1. *Lattice* entered the NMR vocabulary from early studies of solids, in which the extended environment of the nucleus under examination was the orderly, repetitive pattern of atoms in a crystal lattice. Although there is no such orderly lattice structure in liquids, the term has been retained and generalized to include liquids.

We have spoken here of a few intense fluctuations originating nearby, versus a very large number of fluctuations from a distance. This could be compared to the audible noise produced from raindrops on an overhead tin roof versus all the more distant sounds of rain. The individual raindrops striking nearby cause a few discrete, loud sounds, each perceived as an individual event. This is analogous to the few large fluctuations caused by thermal noise originating nearby (the basis of T_2). The sound of distant rain is produced by many raindrops, any one of which is too distant to be audible and which together create a constant hissing sound similar to that of steam escaping. This is analogous to lattice magnetic noise, which contains many frequencies, including the specific frequency stimulating T_1 relaxation.

T_1 AND T_2 IN TISSUES

Each of the factors mentioned above—temperature, paramagnetism, polar macromolecules—changes thermal motion and so alters the magnetic environment of the hydrogen nucleus we are imaging by MRI. Using an NMR relaxation analyzer in a laboratory situation, it is possible to study—in isolation—the effect of each of these factors on the behavior (relaxation times) of the hydrogen nucleus.

Starting with a sample of pure water, there are several things we can do to alter the environment of the nuclei, and so change relaxation time. We can lower the temperature, add an amount of polar macromolecule (protein), or add a paramagnetic substance and then measure the exact changes in T_1 and T_2 independently of each other. Each of the above three factors shortens T_1. Paramagnetic substances also shorten T_2, while adding large molecules or reducing temperature has no effect on T_2. (Temperature is not a significant factor in MRI because the internal temperature of humans is quite constant.) Complex mixtures of liquids can also be analyzed by *in vitro* NMR analysis. T_1 and T_2 of complex mixtures can be measured with considerable accuracy, provided the sample is large enough to be measured, is homogeneous, and enough analysis time is allocated.

Measuring the relaxation times of living tissues using MRI differs substantially from laboratory measurement of simple solutions. First, tissue fluids (particularly inside cells) are very complex mixtures of macromolecules and paramagnetic substances. In addition, the exact composition of tissue fluids at any one moment cannot be determined.

Composition of Tissue Fluids

In pure water, T_1 and T_2 are about equal (2.7 seconds). In tissues, T_1 and T_2 are shorter: T_1 is about one-fifth that of pure water, while T_2 is about one-fiftieth. This shortening of T_1 and T_2 relative to pure water is due to the increased viscosity of tissue water and the presence of paramagnetic substances. The reason for the greater shortening of T_2 relative to T_1 is not clear. It may be that, because magnetically, many cellular components behave as if they were somewhere between a liquid and a solid. In true solids, T_2 is very much shorter than T_1, while T_1 is greatly prolonged. The semi-solid state of much of the tissue hydrogen may explain the absolute T_1 and T_2 observed in tissues. In pathology, changes in the nature of this semi-solid state may explain many of the changes in relaxation times.

Each substance dissolved in tissue water wields its own influence on the behavior of the hydrogen nuclei in the water molecules. The complicated interrelationships between tissue components and their effect on relaxation times are now under intensive study. Much useful data can be expected within the next decade.

Compartmentalization

Another way that T_1 and T_2 measurements of living tissue differ from laboratory measurements is in their lack of homogeneity: except for a few anatomical compartments, such as the cerebral ventricles, amniotic fluid, urinary bladder, cysts, and major vascular channels, large volumes of homogeneous fluid do not occur in the normal body. In living tissues, there is a very complex assemblage of macromolecules, lipoprotein membranes, various intracellular microscopic structures, and paramagnetic substances, which are not homogeneously distributed. Probably, various microscopic cellular compartments have widely differing T_1s and T_2s.

The structure of individual cells can be extremely complex. Each

cell has an endoplasmic reticulum, an extensive labyrinth of pro-
teolipid membrane which has an enormous surface area. Such extensive, relatively stiff, semi-fluid structures probably slow the
movement of adjacent water in the cell cytoplasm and so shorten T_1,
for the same reasons as do dissolved macromolecules. Similarly,
mitochondria, which possess a large area of interfolding membranes, fill up 10–30% of most cells. Both of these highly membranous subcompartments have their own structural and chemical
characteristics and probably differing values for T_1 and T_2. In liver
cells, endoplasmic reticulum and mitochondrial membranes account
for 90% of total tissue membrane (Blouin, Bolender, and Weibel, in
Fawcett, 1981).

An MRI scan consists of thousands of picture elements (pixels).
Each represents a composite of T_1, T_2, and hydrogen distribution
within a particular volume element (voxel) in the body. Scanning
can be weighted to emphasize any one, or a combination, of these
factors. Typical dimensions of a voxel might be $1 \times 1 \times 10$ millimeters. Within this voxel might be several hundred thousand cells,
each with subcompartments having their own T_1 and T_2. Surrounding the cells is a thin layer of extracellular fluid, whose composition
(and therefore T_1 and T_2) is much closer to that of pure water than is
intracellular fluid. (For the entire body, extracellular fluid makes up
an average of 20% of the total tissue volume.) When MRI of living
tissues is performed, the radio signal from the layer of extracellular
fluid surrounding the cells is averaged by the scanner with the signal
from the intracellular water and the various cellular subcompartments, and a composite value results. It will be fascinating to learn,
over the next few years, how microscopic changes in cell membranous structure affect relaxation times in various pathologies.

RELAXATION TIME ACCURACY

In the MRI scanner, it is difficult to take a large enough number
of measurements to provide accurate T_1 and T_2 values, because of
the practical limitations on the length of time the patient can be
expected to lie motionless in the center of the long tube of the MRI
gantry (see Chapter 7). It is difficult to extrapolate from any two or

three image data points to estimate relaxation times accurately. Accuracy would be greatly improved if twenty or thirty data points could be obtained. This is practical in the laboratory but not in the clinical setting. In addition to inconsistencies from a single MRI scanner, relaxation times seem to differ substantially from machine to machine. Greater relaxation time accuracy will undoubtedly be realized in the future.

It is impossible to determine from scans that display T_1 or T_2 just what complex chemical or structural factors have contributed to these relaxation times. In the clinical use of MRI, correlations between pathology and T_1 and T_2 are presently established empirically. For example, while it is known that most types of brain pathological lesions greatly lengthen T_2 (and so are seen best by T_2-weighted scans), the exact reasons for this are not known. While MRI observes hydrogen nuclei and changes in their behavior, it cannot directly observe the macromolecules or paramagnetic substances that cause the environmental changes. All that can be measured in a T_1- or T_2-weighted scan is the *total* change in the magnetic environment affecting these two relaxation times.

To return to the analogy with which we opened this chapter, we can again compare magnetic resonance imaging of hydrogen nuclei to the observation of people on the street below a hotel room window. We know a great deal about human response to weather because of extended, personal observation. We know very little about the behavioral responses of tissue water to different pathophysiological circumstances because we have relatively little experience. It is to be hoped that we will become as familiar with these tissue interrelationships as we are with people responding to the weather.

PULSE-SEQUENCING

Our knowledge of the tissues is derived from the brief signal re-emitted from the tissues after the stimulating pulse. Since both T_1 and T_2 cause the duration of this signal to shorten, how is it possible to distinguish their relative contributions, and produce scans emphasizing either T_1 or T_2?

With the approach to imaging we have described so far—using a single stimulating pulse—it is impossible to separate the effects of

T_1 and T_2. A single pulse gives us an MRI scan displaying mainly regional hydrogen concentration. To measure T_1 and T_2, the stimulation of the tissues is modified. Instead of one pulse of radio frequency energy, two or more pulses are applied in quick succession. Such *pulse-sequences* cause the re-emitted signal to contain information about T_1 and T_2. By changing the parameters of the pulse-sequence—the number of pulses, the strength of the pulses, and the time intervals between the pulses—different types of information can be elicited from the tissues. The MRI scan can be *weighted* to emphasize information about either T_1 or T_2.

When a slice of tissue is scanned using various pulse-sequences, such as spin-echo or inversion-recovery, the resulting scans can appear dramatically different. It is almost as though they were made from large tissue slices actually cut from the organ and stained by various histological techniques (see Figure 8–1). These different pulse-sequences used in MRI are the imaging strategies referred to in Chapter 1. For the interested reader, they will be expanded upon in Chapter 6.

6

Tissue Characterization and Pulse-Sequencing

In preceding chapters, we described the physics of MRI using a classical approach. We started by comparing the properties of a hydrogen nucleus with those of a more familiar object—the compass needle. This comparison was valid because a compass needle and a hydrogen nucleus share several properties. In the presence of a magnetic field, both tend to align with the field, absorb energy through the phenomenon of resonance, and subsequently re-emit this energy. Each oscillates at a frequency proportional to the strength of the magnetic field. In the case of the hydrogen nucleus, this oscillatory frequency is the resonant, or Larmor frequency. To acquire a better understanding of MRI, particularly of tissue characterization and pulse-sequencing, we need to develop a more precise description of nuclear behavior. It would seem logical to start with the study of an individual hydrogen nucleus, just as we started our earlier explanations with the behavior of an individual compass needle. But the detailed description of the behavior of an individual hydrogen nucleus, trillions of times smaller than a compass needle, is extremely complex. Such detailed descriptions require a knowledge of quantum physics and are therefore beyond the scope of this book. (An introduction to quantum principles in MRI is contained in the Appendix.)

Fortunately, it is unnecessary to understand the behavior of a single nucleus in order to understand MRI for, in reality, it is impossible to observe a single nucleus: the signal it generates is much too weak to be measured. What is observed, rather, is the *aggregate* signal from many billions of nuclei. Although individually they obey quantum laws, the collective behavior of the nuclei and the signal they produce can be described in classical terms. The aggregate response of the hydrogen nuclei in the few cubic millimeters of tissue in a voxel is, in many respects, remarkably like one large compass needle.

In modern science, there are many other examples of how detailed knowledge of a process is unnecessary for it to be exploited. A satellite may be put in orbit without any application of the theory of relativity, because the effects of relativity in this particular situation are trivial. Similarly, a motion picture director produces as a final product a developed piece of photographic film but needs know nothing about the theory of the photographic process. In MRI, inclusion of a discussion of the behavior of individual nuclei is not only unnecessary but may also distract from the more relevant consideration of the aggregate behavior of nuclei. In this chapter, we concentrate on the classical description of nuclear behavior, and then apply it to imaging, pulse-sequencing, and T_1- and T_2-weighting of MRI scans.

OSCILLATION OF THE NUCLEUS

Before going on to describe collective behavior, one further comparison between the individual nucleus and the compass needle should be made: their manner of oscillation. Because its movement is restricted by a fixed bearing, a compass needle oscillates in a single plane. The hydrogen nucleus, in three-dimensional space, oscillates in a wobbling motion about the direction of the magnetic field. This type of motion is called *precession*. We are familiar with it as the wobbling motion of a spinning toy top in the earth's gravitational field. (The earth itself wobbles about its axis in the same manner.) The number of times per second that the nucleus wobbles or precesses about the field direction is its resonant frequency (Figure 6–1).

Toward the end of the nineteenth century, English physicist Joseph Larmor described the precessional motion atomic particles exhibit when placed in a magnetic field. The frequency of precession is called the *Larmor frequency*. This precessional motion is a gen-

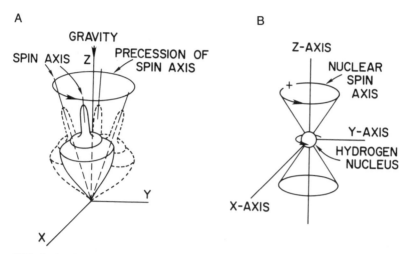

FIG. 6–1. The toy top (**A**) spins about its own axis, which precesses in the earth's gravitational field. The hydrogen nucleus (**B**) possesses nuclear spin; its spin axis precesses in the magnetic field of the scanner.

eral phenomenon, exhibited for example by electrons. The precession of the hydrogen nucleus in nuclear magnetic resonance is but one example.

THE MAGNETIZATION VECTOR

To describe the behavior of hydrogen nuclei during MRI, we use an imaginary construct: the *magnetization vector*, a single arrow that represents the aggregate behavior of all hydrogen nuclei in a small region of tissue. While most texts use the magnetization vector to represent an "infinitely small region" of tissue, for convenience we will say that this small region is a voxel, the volume element of tissue being imaged. The magnetization vector is described using a coordinate system whose X, Y, and Z axes coincide with those of the scanner's magnetic field and whose origin is in the middle of the voxel of tissue being imaged. The tail of the vector is fixed at this origin, and its length and direction at any moment express the overall behavior of the hydrogen nuclei in the voxel.

The magnetization vector may usefully be compared to a weather vane. Air atoms move with a frenetic random motion, on average at about the speed of sound. Many millions of air atoms strike the weather vane each second. In still air, the number of such impacts on all surfaces of the vane is nearly constant; they cancel each other, and the vane points in no particular direction. In a wind, the molecules continue this random motion, but in addition, the atoms exhibit a much slower net motion in a particular direction. The weathervane expresses this net motion, ignoring the random. From moment to moment, the direction of the weathervane changes to reflect changes in wind direction (Figure 6–2). Similarly, in tissues, there is a very large number of water molecules undergoing random thermal motion. When there is no external magnetic field, the nuclear orientations are randomly directed, much as the movement of air atoms in still air. In MRI, the nuclei are exposed to the additional influences of the constant magnetic fields of the scanner and intermittent radio energy. When the nuclei are exposed to a constant magnetic field, they have a small net tendency to align with this field. When exposed to radio energy, they have a small net tendency to be driven away from alignment. The magnetization vector ex-

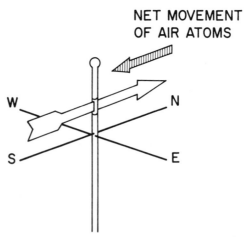

FIG. 6–2. A weathervane indicates the net movement of air molecules, even though they are all moving randomly at about the speed of sound. In tissues, the magnetization vector represents the net behavior of the nuclei in the randomly moving molecules; the nuclei tend to align with the scanner's magnetic field.

presses the average magnetic orientation of the nuclei in the voxel under examination at any moment, in response to these influences, in the same way that the weathervane expresses changes in atmospheric conditions.

The behavior of the magnetization vector represents non-random forces and movements of the nuclei in the voxel. In the applied external magnetic field of the MRI scanner, the non-random forces are really a very small fraction of the total forces in a voxel. Even in MRI scanners with the strongest main fields, most of the motion of the nuclei is dominated by random thermal motion, the basis of Brownian movement. This vector allows us to make the conceptual leap from the magnetic behavior of a compass needle to the aggre-

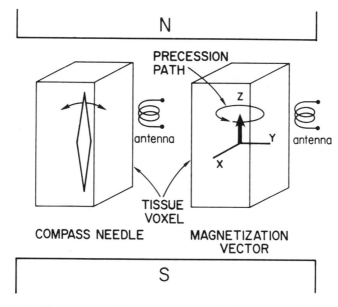

FIG. 6–3. When energized, a compass needle in a magnetic field oscillates in a plane, inducing a signal in an antenna coil. The magnetic behavior of the many hydrogen nuclei in a voxel of tissue can be represented by a single arrow, the magnetization vector. In many ways, this vector behaves as if it were a real bar magnet, such as a compass needle. When it absorbs energy, it oscillates in a precessional motion about the Z-axis, inducing a signal in the antenna.

gate behavior of many magnetic nuclei in tissues. Although individually, nuclei must be described by quantum physics, their aggregate behavior can be expressed by the magnetization vector, which is described classically, in a manner more analogous to a compass needle. For teaching purposes, we can substitute the magnetization vector for the compass needle in many of our earlier explanations (Figure 6–3).

General Behavior of the Magnetization Vector

This section describes, in a general manner, the behavior of the magnetization vector during the MRI scan process: alignment before stimulation, stimulation by radio-frequency energy, oscillation, and subsequent loss of energy.

When a patient is placed in the strong magnetic field of an MRI scanner, hydrogen nuclei in the tissues tend to align themselves with the field: the magnetization vector reflects this by aligning with the main field of the scanner (along the positive Z-axis). The length of the vector is proportional both to the number of nuclei in the voxel and to the applied magnetic field strength. When the voxel of tissue is exposed to radio frequency energy (at the Larmor frequency), the nuclei absorb energy and tend to deflect away from alignment with the main field; the magnetization vector deflects so that it tilts away from the direction of the main field. Just as the angle to which a compass needle is deflected depends on how hard it has been tapped, so too, the angle to which the magnetization vector tilts is proportional to the strength of the radio-frequency pulse.

Once energized, the tilted magnetization vector precesses about the Z-axis at the Larmor frequency, representing an extremely large number of individually precessing nuclei. The angle that the precessing magnetization vector makes with the main field gradually diminishes; eventually the vector comes back to rest aligned with the main field. This represents the behavior of the nuclei as they lose energy and tend to come back into alignment with the main field.

Magnetization Vector and Signal

For the purposes of MRI, the magnetization vector can be treated as if it were a real magnet. When a real magnet moves in relation to a stationary antenna coil, its lines of magnetic force cut through the coil, inducing a voltage. In MRI, the magnetization vector is at rest before stimulation, lying along the positive Z-axis; at this time it induces no voltage in the antenna coil. After stimulation, the vector is in motion, precessing about the positive Z-axis. As it does so, the vector (like a bar magnet) induces in the antenna of the MRI scanner an oscillating signal; the frequency of this signal is the Larmor frequency.

In the imaging process, all the voxels in the slice of tissue being imaged are stimulated: the magnetization vector for each voxel is tipped away from the Z-axis by the same angle. Initially, the vectors all precess at the same Larmor frequency. But to furthur localize the voxels, the scanner applies a new gradient transversely across the slice, slightly raising or lowering the magnetic field at various locations in the slice (see Chapter 4: Imaging). In response, the Larmor frequency of the magnetization vector for each voxel changes accordingly, so that the vectors at different locations in the slice induce signals of different frequencies in the antenna. The position of a voxel in the gradient can thus be deduced from the frequency of its signal.

A recognition of the immediate responses of the magnetization vector to changes in local field strength following excitation is crucial to the understanding of MRI. In the next section, the magnetization vector is considered in more detail. This will provide insight into T_1, T_2, and signal strength.

COMPONENT VECTORS

Most mathematical descriptions of a vector in three-dimensional space describe the vector as a sum of three component vectors, one for each of the coordinate axes—X, Y, and Z. By summing the components lying along each of the axes, a vector of any length and orientation can be obtained. A simple example of the addition of vectors is the points of a compass (Figure 6–4).

In MRI, it is convenient to describe the magnetization vector in terms of only two component vectors. One vector lies on the Z-axis, parallel to the main field, which runs head-to-foot in the patient. The second vector lies in the plane defined by the X- and Y-axes, at right angles to the main field (Figure 6–5). This second vector

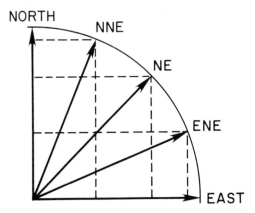

FIG. 6–4. A single vector can be expressed as the sum of two (or three) vectors. For example, the points of a compass can be expressed as the sum of any two cardinal directions. Northeast, for instance, is the sum of equal-length vectors pointing in the north and east directions.

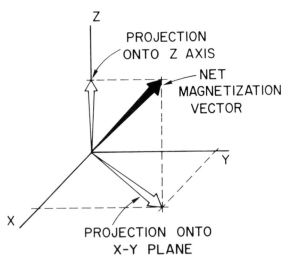

FIG. 6–5. The length of the magnetization vector is proportional to the number of hydrogen nuclei in the voxel. At any moment during imaging, the direction of the vector indicates the average position of these nuclei. Here the magnetization vector is shown tipped 45° from the Z-axis, toward the X-Y plane. Its longitudinal and transverse projections (onto the Z-axis and the X-Y plane respectively) are equal.

could be further resolved as the sum of vectors along the X- and Y-axes, similar to compass points. Since the main field in most scanners is longitudinal, the Z-axis component is usually referred to as the *longitudinal* component, while the vector in the X-Y plane is the *transverse* component. (By convention, the Y-axis is front-to-back of the patient, X-axis is left-to-right.)

The importance of the components of the magnetization vector is that each is related to an aspect of nuclear behavior: the longitudinal component is related to T_1, and the transverse component to T_2. We will see that the transverse component is also related to signal strength. With these simple tools, we can describe in a more precise manner the response of the magnetization vector to a radio frequency pulse.

Components of the Magnetization Vector after Stimulation

Before stimulation, the magnetization vector is entirely longitudinal, being aligned with the main field along the positive Z-axis. It is stationary, has no transverse component, and produces no signal. Upon stimulation, the magnetization vector is driven away from the positive Z-axis, resulting in the longitudinal and transverse components' taking on new values. In MRI, the strength of the stimulating pulse is indicated by the number of degrees it deflects the magnetization vector: for example, 10°, 45°, 90°, 180° are some of the pulse strengths used. Because the length of the magnetization vector is the same immediately after stimulation as before, the initial values of its longitudinal and transverse components are determined by the exact angle to which the magnetization vector is driven. For example, with a relatively short (weak) pulse, the vector might be deflected only 10°. As a result, the longitudinal vector shortens slightly, while the transverse vector attains a small, but measurable value.

Using pulses of increasing strength, from zero to 90°, results in shorter longitudinal components and longer transverse components. A 90° pulse places the magnetization vector entirely in the transverse plane, producing the maximum length transverse component, and a length of zero for the longitudinal component. Increasing pulse strengths from 90° to 180° results in a shorter transverse component, but also in a longitudinal component that is longer in the negative (downward, or caudal) Z-axis direction. At 180°, the longitudinal component achieves a maximum negative value, while the transverse component becomes zero. Still stronger pulses drive the magnetization vector beyond 180°, producing a longitudinal component that is shorter in the negative Z-direction, but a transverse component that is larger. At 270°, the longitudinal component is zero, while the transverse component is again maximal. Similarly, pulses between 270° and 360° produce longitudinal components that are longer in the positive Z-direction, and transverse components that are again shorter. At 360°, the magnetization vector is driven completely around a circle, coming to rest in the positive Z direction, in its pre-stimulation state.

With the exception of 180° and 360° pulses (which place the magnetization vector along the negative and positive Z-axis, respectively), the magnetization vector is tilted away from the Z-axis, and precesses at the Larmor frequency.

Transverse Component and Signal Strength

There are several reasons to analyze the magnetization vector in terms of its component vectors. The first of these concerns signal strength.

Earlier we stated that the precessing magnetization vector induces a measurable signal in the antenna coil. The antenna of the MRI scanner essentially consists of a pair of coils of wire lying perpendicular to the X-Y plane. Only the component of the magnetic vector's precessional motion that is at right angles to the antenna (i.e., the transverse component) can induce this voltage. *Therefore, the signal strength from a voxel is proportional to the length of the transverse component.*

We saw earlier that the stimulating radio-frequency pulse drives the magnetization vectors for all the voxels in the slice of tissue being imaged to approximately the same angle, where they precess at a Larmor frequency appropriate to their position in the transverse gradient. We know that the length of an individual magnetization vector depends on the number of hydrogen nuclei in its voxel: the more nuclei in a voxel, the longer its magnetization vector. This in turn results in a longer transverse component, and a stronger signal from that voxel. The length of the magnetization vector also increases when stronger external field strengths are used, as in high-field MRI scanners. In such high-field strengths, the magnetization vector induces a stronger signal in the X-Y receiving antenna. Since the noise (mostly thermal noise from the patient) remains constant, the signal-to-noise ratio is better in a stronger field.

The antenna measures the signal from a slice of tissue after a single excitation pulse; in the presence of a transverse gradient, the antenna receives signals at many slightly different frequencies. Each frequency component of this signal corresponds to the position of a line across the slice of tissue in the gradient. The strength of the signal at that frequency indicates the number of nuclei in that line of tissue. This information can then be used to create images. (See Chapter 4: Imaging.)

Component Vectors and Tissue Characterization

The initial length of the transverse component (and the initial signal strength from a voxel) is an indication of regional tissue hydrogen concentration. But in MRI, we are interested in tissue characterization beyond simple hydrogen concentration: specifically, the rate at which nuclei lose energy (T_1) and the rate at which nuclei become dephased (T_2). To determine T_1 and T_2, we must examine the behavior of the magnetization vector's components after stimulation, as the nuclei relax back to their pre-stimulation state. To measure T_1, we must examine how rapidly the longitudinal component changes; to analyze T_2, we must measure the rate at which the transverse component disappears.

While the above discussion focused mainly on the initial lengths of the transverse and longitudinal vectors immediately after stimulation, it is the subsequent behavior of these vectors—how they change after stimulation—that reflects tissue characteristics. The next section considers the behavior of the transverse and longitudinal components as expressions of T_1 and T_2.

BEHAVIOR OF LONGITUDINAL AND
TRANSVERSE COMPONENTS

Because T_1 and T_2 are largely independent processes, we must conceptualize the behavior of the longitudinal and transverse components of the magnetization vector separately. We can then use these component vectors to compare the rates T_1 and T_2, and to relate these relaxation processes to signal strength.

Longitudinal Component and T_1

The longitudinal vector is related to the energy of the nuclei in the voxel; the initial length and orientation of the longitudinal component immediately after stimulation is related to the amount of energy absorbed by the nuclei; the rate at which the longitudinal vector changes length after stimulation expresses how rapidly energy is lost from the nuclei. (This is expressed as the time constant T_1.)

Before stimulation, the magnetization vector is entirely longitudinal, lying at rest along the positive Z-axis. As stated above, the initial length of the longitudinal component after stimulation is related to the angle to which the magnetization vector is driven, which in turn is related to the amount of energy in the stimulating pulse: the longitudinal component takes on some value between its original extreme length in the positive (up) Z direction, and the same length in the negative (down) Z direction. (In Figure 6–6, the magnetization vector is shown before and after a 180° pulse.)

After stimulation, the nuclei start to lose their energy; the longitudinal component starts to return upward in the positive Z direction. The rate of energy loss, as well as the rate at which the longitudinal component grows upward, is determined by T_1. No matter what its initial length and orientation after stimulation (whether directed along the positive or negative Z-axis), the longitudinal component starts to grow back in the positive Z direction at rate T_1 (Figure 6–7). The upward growth of the longitudinal component (which indicates T_1 energy loss) cannot be measured directly, because the MRI scanner's antenna can measure only the transverse component. But it can be measured indirectly, using the spin-echo

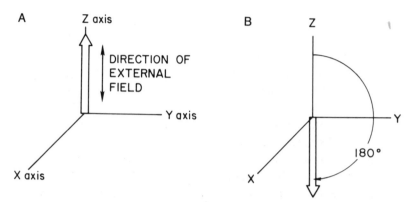

FIG. 6–6. A: Before stimulation the positive (upward) longitudinal component is maximal. **B:** After a 180° pulse, the longitudinal component has the same length but lies along the negative Z-axis.

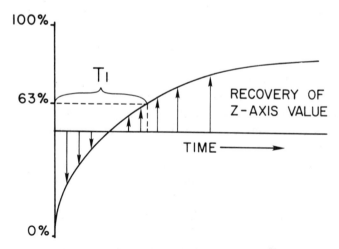

FIG. 6–7. The growth of the longitudinal component after a 180° pulse is shown. After a stimulating pulse, the nuclei undergo T_1 relaxation (energy loss) at an exponential rate. T_1 is defined as the time it takes for the longitudinal component to regain 63% of its length.

and inversion-recovery pulse sequences. Both are described later in this chapter.

There seems to be a paradox concerning the relationship between the amount of energy in the stimulating pulse and the length of time it takes the longitudinal component to regain its original state. In general, the more energy that is contained in the stimulating radio pulse, the larger the angle through which the magnetization vector is deflected. As pulse strength increases from zero to 180°, the longitudinal component becomes longer in the negative Z direction, and it takes longer for the longitudinal component to return to its original positive Z orientation. So far, this seems logical: the more energy "pumped" into the tissues, the longer it takes for the tissues to dissipate the energy, and the longer it takes the longitudinal component to return to equilibrium. But at pulses stronger than 180°, the relationship between the energizing pulse and the longitudinal component becomes counter-intuitive: the pulses contain more energy, but result in a longitudinal component that is shorter, and that takes less time to grow back to its pre-stimulation state. Although seemingly illogical, this behavior has its roots in quantum physics, and must be accepted in order to develop an understanding of MRI.

Transverse Component

After a stimulating radio frequency pulse, the magnetic vector has a measurable transverse component (except when the stimulating pulse is 180° or 360°). Because it is precessing at the Larmor frequency, the transverse component is an expression of the precessional motion of the nuclei within the voxel. The length of the transverse component at any moment after stimulation is an expression of the phase coherence between the nuclei, that is, how well their phases are locked together.

The stimulating radio-frequency pulse locks in phase the precessional motions of the nuclei in the voxel: immediately after excitation, the transverse component of the magnetization vector has a maximum length and is precessing at the Larmor frequency. Although the nuclei are initially locked in phase by the stimulating pulse, local randomly changing forces in the tissue cause fluctuations in the precessional rate of individual nuclei: the nuclei quickly become dephased. As their phase relationships become random, the nuclei cancel each other's magnetic effects: the transverse component shrinks and disappears. Because it is both shortening and rotating, the tip of the transverse component describes an ever-narrowing spiral. When the nuclei are completely dephased, the transverse component is zero. The rate at which the transverse component changes length (shortens) expresses the rate of dephasing (T_2).

Sources of Dephasing: T_2 and T_2-star

There are two important causes of dephasing. The first, T_2 from thermal motion in tissues, was discussed in Chapter 5 because of its importance in characterizing tissues. The second, non-uniformity of the field strength, is presented here for the first time.

Non-uniformity of field is actually the major source of dephasing in MRI. Due to inevitable, constant non-uniformities in the scanner's magnetic field, tissue magnetic properties, and applied gradient fields, there are slight but important variations in field strength from point to point within the volume being imaged. Since they are fixed, these non-uniformities are fundamentally different from those fluctuations that occur due to random thermal motion (described in Chapter 5). The term for dephasing due to fixed distortions of the field is T_2-star. Although it does not reflect tissue characteristics, T_2-star nonetheless plays an important role in the imaging process.

The Sources of T_2-star

No magnet can produce a perfectly uniform magnetic field. Although the magnets used in MRI create magnetic fields that are extremely uniform (from one part in ten thousand to one in a million), even such slight imperfections can have striking effects. Two adjacent anatomical regions may differ in field strength by only one part in a million, but if their precessional frequency is 50 million cycles per second, they will drift 180° out of phase in ten milliseconds. This indicates the importance of the effects of even slight field non-uniformity.

The field of the scanner is also distorted by the presence of the patient's body, which has very weak magnetic properties. To understand this, we can think how a piece of iron placed in a uniform magnetic field will attract and concentrate the magnetic field within itself, causing the field strength there to be much greater than elsewhere. This ability to concentrate the magnetic field is called *magnetic susceptibility*. To a much less striking degree than iron, various regions of tissue have varying magnetic susceptibility, resulting in different field strengths within an initially uniform field. This can come, for example, from paramagnetic atoms found in varying quantities in the tissues. In the presence of the scanner's magnetic field, these become aligned, causing a slight, unpredictable regional concentration of the main field. (Even if one could produce a perfectly uniform field, placing a patient in the field destroys this uniformity, and in a manner peculiar to each patient.)

In addition to these uncontrollable non-uniformities, there is the intentionally created non-uniformity due to the magnetic gradients. In our explanations up to now, we have assumed that an individual voxel is exposed to a uniform field. In fact, the gradient creates a differential magnetic field across the voxel. In practice, the gradient magnetic fields usually are the strongest of these three sources of dephasing. All three sources of non-uniformity of field are constant over time and cause the Larmor frequency to vary slightly in different regions of the field. As a result, the precessional phase relationships of the nuclei drift apart in a constant and predictable manner.

The dephasing of hydrogen nuclei, then, comes from these constant sources of non-uniformity, as well as from the fluctuating non-uniformities due to the tissues' random thermal magnetic noise. In practice, the dephasing caused by constant non-uniformities of field (T_2-star) contributes much more dephasing than that caused by thermal noise (T_2). There is an important difference between the dephasing produced by T_2 and that produced by T_2-star: constant non-uniformities cause nuclei to go out of phase with each other at a constant rate (T_2-star); but random fluctuations from thermal noise cause nuclei to go out of phase randomly (T_2).

Dephasing and Signal Strength

Immediately after excitation, the transverse component of the magnetization vector is long, signifying that the precessional phase coherence is high. Precessions are not cancelling other nearby precessions but instead reinforce each other; consequently, the received radio signal is strong. As the nuclei go out of phase, the transverse component shortens and the signal weakens. While the initial amplitude of the signal is a measure of hydrogen concentration, the rate of decay of the signal indicates the rate of dephasing due to T_2 and T_2-star.

ROTATING FRAME OF REFERENCE

Until now, we have been observing the motion of the transverse component from a stationary, external point of view. We see it rotating at the Larmor frequency about the Z-axis, as it shortens due to dephasing. To simplify analysis of this process, it is common to imagine that the point of view of the observer is some distance above the transverse plane, on the Z-axis, and rotating at approximately the Larmor frequency. This is called the *rotating frame of reference*.

Because our frame of reference is rotating with the transverse component, the magnetization vector lying in the transverse plane appears stationary, and minor changes in phase relationships can be observed with great precision. When using the magnetization vector to describe nuclear behavior, it is necessary to specify whether the frame of reference is external (stationary) or rotating (Figure 6–8). This means of examining rotating objects could be illustrated by a merry-go-round. If we stand outside the merry-go-round and observe its motion, as the various horses and other objects blur past us, we could not distinguish any of their details. However, if we climbed to the top and looked through a hole on the axis of rotation, we would be turning with the entire array of horses and passengers; each of them would now seem to be nearly stationary, and we could tell one horse from another and even recognize passengers. By rotating with this complicated machine, we place ourselves in its frame of reference.

We can examine the effect of a pulse on the magnetization vector, and the subsequent behavior of the vector as viewed from a rotating frame of reference. But before doing so, we should point out two facts about radio-pulse/tissue interaction. First, in MRI, radio-fre-

A   B

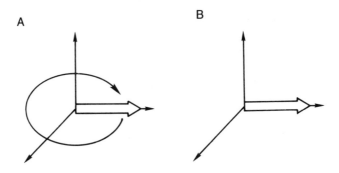

FIG. 6–8. A: The magnetization vector after a 90° pulse, as viewed from an external frame. The vector lies in the transverse plane, and rotates at the larmor frequency. **B:** The magnetization vector after a 90° pulse, as viewed from a rotating frame. The vector appears to lie still in the transverse plane. It is easier to use the magnetization vector in the rotating frame to describe subtle changes in subsequent precessional motion.

quency pulses arrive from a specific direction (usually along the X-axis) and are not simply beamed into the tissues from all sides. Second, when the magnetization vector is deflected by the pulse, it tends to align perpendicularly to the direction of the radio-frequency pulse.

Consider a 90° pulse entering the tissues in the transverse plane along the X-axis. The magnetization vector, which is originally aligned with the upward positive Z-axis, is deflected 90° into the X-Y plane, and lies along the Y-axis (perpendicular to the direction of origin of the pulse). Initially, the transverse magnetization vector appears as a single vector, because the nuclei are in phase. Because we are rotating with it (at the Larmor frequency), it appears to lie stationary on the Y-axis. As time passes and the precessional rates of nuclei change, we observe the transverse component dispersing into many shorter vectors in the X-Y plane, fanning out clockwise and counterclockwise away from the original Y-axis transverse component, thereby expressing the fact that nuclei are drifting ahead or behind in phase (Figure 6–9). In this rotating frame of

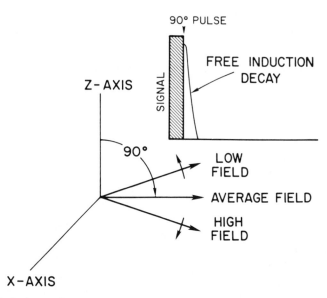

FIG. 6–9. Immediately after the stimulating pulse, the nuclei are precessing in phase. But due to non-uniformities in the field, they precess at different rates, becoming progressively dephased. As seen in the rotating frame, the transverse component disperses into many vectors, which spread clockwise and counterclockwise in the X-Y plane.

reference, we could also distinguish the two sources of dephasing: that due to constant, local, field non-uniformities (T_2-star) and that due to randomly changing thermal motion (T_2): the vectors representing T_2-star dephasing fan out at constant rates, while those representing T_2 dephasing spread out randomly.

Understanding the rotating frame of reference and this particular example (the 90° pulse) will be important to understanding the spin-echo pulse-sequence, to be covered later in this chapter.

COMPARING THE LONGITUDINAL AND
TRANSVERSE COMPONENTS

In summary, the magnetization vector expresses, in a single arrow, the average non-random behavior of hydrogen nuclei in a region of tissue. By noting its projections onto the longitudinal Z-axis or onto the transverse X-Y plane, we can examine more specific behavior: the growing projection on the Z-axis describes T_1 relaxation; the shrinking projection on the X-Y plane describes T_2 and T_2-star relaxation. As an example, consider the stimulation of nuclei in a voxel by a 90° pulse. Using the longitudinal and transverse components, we will compare the rates of energy loss and dephasing, and then correlate this behavior with the measured signal.

Before stimulation, the magnetization vector is entirely longitudinal, has a finite value, and points upward along the positive Z-axis; the transverse component is zero. In this unstimulated equilibrium state, there is no signal being produced. The tissue is exposed to a 90° pulse; the pulse drives the magnetization vector 90° into the transverse plane, putting the precessions of the nuclei into phase with each other. The longitudinal component is zero immediately after this stimulation, but the length of the transverse component is maximal, and it rotates in the X-Y plane at the Larmor frequency (as viewed from the stationary external frame of reference), thereby inducing a signal in the antenna coil (Figure 6–10). The nuclei immediately begin to lose their energy (due to T_1) and their precessional motions start to become dephased (due to T_2 and T_2-star); the longitudinal component begins to grow in the positive Z direction, while at the same time the transverse component begins to shrink toward zero (Figure 6–11).

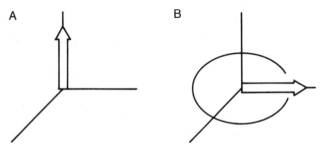

FIG. 6–10. A: A 90° pulse tilts the magnetization vector from its original longitudinal orientation, into the transverse plane. **B:** In a stationary frame, the magnetization vector rotates in the transverse plane at the Larmor frequency.

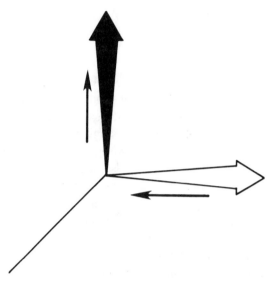

FIG. 6–11. As viewed from a rotating frame, the transverse component shortens (at a rate determined by dephasing) and the longitudinal component grows (at a rate determined by energetic loss). Dephasing occurs more rapidly than energetic loss, so shortening of the transverse component occurs more rapidly than growth of the longitudinal component. As the transverse component shortens, the detected signal decays. The *black arrow* shows the final equilibrium position of the vector after complete relaxation.

In tissues, dephasing occurs much more rapidly than T_1 energy loss: T_2 is 20–120 milliseconds, T_2-star is 1–10 milliseconds, while T_1 is between 150 and 2,000 milliseconds. Consequently, the transverse component, under the influence of T_2-star, shortens faster than the longitudinal component, diminishing to zero in perhaps 10 milliseconds, long before the longitudinal component regains its original length. The loss of signal is correspondingly rapid. By the time the transverse component reaches zero, the longitudinal component has regained only a fraction of its original length. The longitudinal component continues to grow, at a rate T_1, until it reaches its original (pre-stimulation) length and orientation. This fact—that the signal falls to zero long before T_1 energy loss is complete—will be important in discussions of the spin-echo pulse-sequence (later in this chapter), and of scan time (in Chapter 9).

PULSE STRENGTH, SIGNAL STRENGTH, AND SIGNAL LOSS

We wish to measure T_1 and T_2, but these relaxation times are impossible to measure using a single pulse. T_1 cannot be measured because the longitudinal component produces no signal. Similarly, T_2 alone cannot be measured, because its dephasing effects are combined with those of T_2-star. Using a single pulse, the only information we can gain from tissues is hydrogen concentration. To measure T_1 or T_2 alone, we must use pulse-sequencing.

A pulse-sequence consists of a series of several pulses of different strengths, separated by different time intervals. Before discussing pulse-sequencing, however, we need to consider in more detail tissue response to a single radio-frequency pulse, the topic of previous sections. Specifically, we will investigate the relationships between pulse strength, signal strength, and signal loss.

Apparatus

To simplify our presentation, we will use a simple apparatus similar to that used by Bloch and by Purcell to demonstrate the phenomenon of NMR in 1946. It consists of a strong permanent magnet between whose pole faces is suspended a small test tube, which contains a small sample representing our tissue voxel. Around this test tube there are two loops of wire: One loop transmits the stimulating radio signal into the sample; the other loop is an antenna measuring the subsequent signal-out from the sample (Figure 6–12). By connecting the antenna to a radio receiver and displaying the output signal on an oscilloscope, we can observe in detail the answer to each question—the shape and amplitude of the emitted signal.

In these experiments, the sample is exposed to a uniform field so that all the hydrogens in the sample experience approximately the same field strength and have the same Larmor frequency. If the test tube is exposed to a 1 tesla field, the resonant Larmor frequency of the hydrogen in the sample is 42.6 million cycles per second. In the following basic experiments, the radio signal used to stimulate the sample has this frequency.

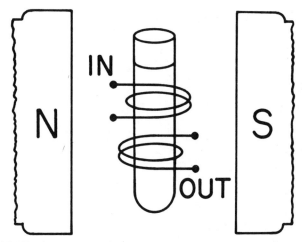

FIG. 6–12. To demonstrate the "response" of a tissue sample to magnetic "interrogation," only a simple apparatus is needed. A test tube is placed between the poles of a magnet. Two loops of wire encircle the test tube, one transmitting a short burst of radio-frequency energy into the sample, the other acting as an antenna that listens to the signal emitted by the sample (in this case blood serum).

The sample in the test-tube is blood serum, which is almost entirely water. (It is the magnetic environment of these water molecules we are analyzing.) Various dissolved substances cause it to behave less like pure water, and more like tissue.

The Free-Induction Decay Signal

In this experiment, we expose the test-tube sample to a single pulse and observe the re-emitted signal immediately after the pulse. If the pulse length is 180° or 360°, there will be no measurable signal (because there is no transverse component). But after pulses of other lengths, there is a transverse component, and a signal can be detected; the sample re-emits the energy in a smoothly decaying signal. This signal is called the *free-induction decay*. This brief, decaying signal is the sole source of information from which images can be constructed (Figure 6–13).

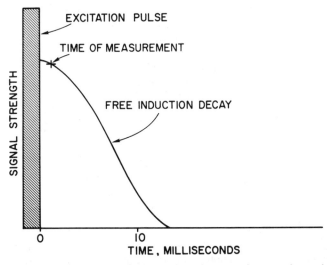

FIG. 6–13. After a single excitation pulse, the sample re-emits a signal of the same frequency as the original excitation pulse. The signal is measured shortly after excitation, near its maximum, and falls to zero within a few milliseconds. This free induction decay signal contains the information for MRI image formation.

Responses to Pulses of Varying Strength

In the next experiment, we expose the sample to pulses of increasing duration/strength, and observe the effects on the amplitude of the re-emitted signal. In MRI, pulse strength is increased not by using a more powerful transmitter, but by using pulses of longer duration. In this experiment, we expose the sample to pulses of increasing duration.

Each pulse is followed by a signal that decays quickly, but smoothly. Here, we are not concerned with the shape of the decaying signal but with its amplitude, which is maximal immediately following the pulse. If we compared the initial amplitude of the signal following each pulse, we would see a striking effect. As we increase the pulse length starting from zero, the amplitude of the signal rises, becoming maximal at some particular pulse duration (here, arbitrarily at 10 microseconds). It then begins to decrease, falling to zero at 20 microseconds—twice the duration of the pulse producing the maximum. As the pulses are made still longer, another maximum is found at 30 microseconds, and another zero reading at 40 microseconds (Figure 6–14).

Why this peculiar relationship should exist between the length of the excitation pulse and the amplitude of the subsequent decaying signal is not immediately apparent but can be understood using the magnetization vector.

Earlier in this chapter we described the relationship between the magnetization vector and signal strength. The magnetization vector expresses the response of all the magnetic nuclei in a voxel to stimulating radio pulses: a radio pulse drives the magnetization vector away from the positive Z-axis by a number of degrees proportional to the strength of the pulse. Its projections on the longitudinal Z-axis and the transverse X-Y plane depend on the angle to which the magnetization vector is driven. The longitudinal component cannot be measured directly, but the transverse component is directly related to signal strength: the longer the transverse component, the stronger will be the received signal. Although we might think that

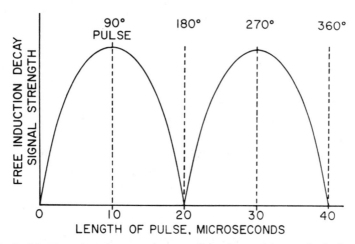

FIG. 6–14. Exposing the sample to radio pulses of increasingly longer length results in remarkable changes in the amplitude of the free induction decay signal. Two maxima and three minima are observed: the maxima at 90° and 270°, and the minima at zero, 180° and 360°.

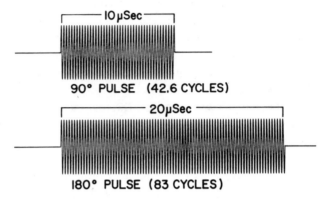

O.I T FIELD STRENGTH, HYDROGEN EXCITATION

10 µSec

90° PULSE (42.6 CYCLES)

20µSec

180° PULSE (83 CYCLES)

FIG. 6–15. The strength of the pulse is determined by its length and intensity. In a given field strength, with a transmitter of fixed power output, a 180° pulse is twice as long as a 90° pulse.

applying more energy to tissues would increase signal output, this is not the case: only the transverse component of the magnetization vector induces a signal. The graph in Figure 6–14 represents the change in length of the transverse component as the magnetization vector is rotated through 360°. In this particular example, the maximum length of the transverse component (and maximum signal strength) occurs at pulse lengths of 10 and 30 microseconds, representing 90° and 180° pulses. Minimum transverse component length (and zero signal strength) occurs at 20 and 40 microseconds, representing 180° and 360° pulses.

With this apparatus, the duration of the 90° pulse is actually determined by the sample size and transmitter power. Because a strong transmitter was used with a very small sample, the duration of the pulse needed to tip the magnetization vector of the sample was short—in the microsecond range. A weaker transmitter, or a larger sample, would require a pulse of longer duration to tip the magnetization vector 90° (Figure 6–15). In clinical MRI scanners, the excitation transmitter can generate about 10,000 watts of power. Because the volume of tissue is very large, the duration of the 90° pulse might be in the range of 1–5 milliseconds. How much radio-frequency power is needed to tip the vector 90° or 180° varies from patient to patient: the pulses must be tuned before each patient is examined, in order to tailor the pulse power to the volume of tissue to be excited.

Signal Loss and Relaxation Times

The initial amplitude of the signal depends on the strength of the pulse. Regardless of the initial amplitude of the free-induction decay, the shape of the decay curve is always similar. The decay of the signal is caused by the relaxation processes: T_1, T_2, and T_2-star. In normal soft tissues, T_1 is 150–2,000 milliseconds, T_2 is 30–120 milliseconds, while T_2-star is 5–15 milliseconds. Comparing these relaxation times, we can see that T_2-star contributes the most to observed signal decay: the free-induction decay signal falls to zero in 5–10 milliseconds. T_2 also contributes significantly to signal loss during these 5–10 milliseconds, but the slight effect of T_1 can be ignored (Figure 6–16).

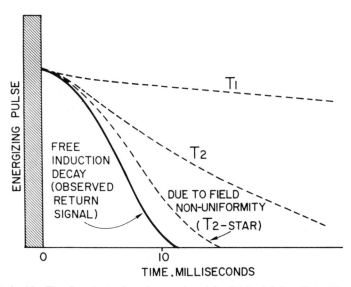

FIG. 6–16. The free induction decay signal (*solid line*) falls off rapidly, under the influence of three factors: energetic decay (T_1), dephasing due to thermal motion (T_2), and dephasing due to field non-uniformity (T_2-star). The dashed lines indicate the separate influence of each factor. T_2-star is the dominant source of signal loss.

The decay of the signal after a single pulse—the free-induction decay—is caused primarily by T_2 and T_2-star dephasing. It is T_2 that we wish to measure, but, since its effect on the free-induction decay is mixed with that of T_2-star, the free-induction decay produced by single-pulse imaging cannot be used to measure T_2 alone. This is one reason for developing pulse-sequencing. In the next section, we see how it is possible, through the spin-echo pulse-sequence, to use T_2-star to measure T_2. Another pulse-sequence—inversion-recovery—can provide T_1 information.

PULSE-SEQUENCING

MRI is magnetic interrogation of tissues: We ask a question of the tissues, listen to the body's answer, and analyze the response. The question we ask is in the form of radio-frequency energy, and the answer is in the form of the free-induction radio-frequency decay signal measured subsequently by the antenna. Coded into the signal is information about tissue properties. Understanding MRI image formation becomes a matter of understanding the relationships between the stimulating radio-frequency question and the tissue's answer.

In the last section, we discussed, using the magnetization vector, the body's response to a single pulse, which is the simplest possible question; the smoothly decaying signal emitted from the tissues after the pulse is the simplest possible answer. The question this single pulse asks is "What is the regional concentration of hydrogen?" The signal emitted by the tissues contains the answer to this question, because the amplitude of the signal produced by each voxel of tissue indicates its hydrogen content: an MRI scan based on a single pulse is largely a map of the distribution of hydrogen in the body. In practice, such an image is of limited diagnostic value.

However, modern MRI asks more complex questions; usually, further tissue characterization is desired, including regional T_1 and T_2, and blood flow. These cannot be obtained using a single pulse; instead, pulse-sequencing is used: a series of two or more radio pulses applied to the tissues in quick succession. The use of a pulse-sequence to stimulate the tissues results in a quite different type of signal from the tissues. This signal contains information about tissue T_1 and T_2 because the tissue's response to later pulses is determined by earlier pulses in the sequence. A further elaboration of the pulse-sequence can be made by repeating it after a lapse of time: The tissue is exposed to several rapid bursts of energy and, after a longer pause, to an identical series of rapid bursts.

This repetition of the pulse-sequence can provide still more tissue characterization. A specific pulse-sequence is defined by the timing between individual pulses, and between clusters of pulses. In general, there is first a tissue "preparation pulse" that sets the stage for the "read" pulse (or pulses). *The free-induction decay after the first pulse exists for only a few milliseconds but the much slower T_1 and T_2 relaxations continue in the absence of a detectable signal.*

Depending on the information we seek, the question asked by the pulse-sequence must be phrased in a specific form. Factors affecting the formulation of the question include: (1) What region of the body is being examined, and (2) What information is to be elicited (hydrogen distribution, T_1, T_2, or blood flow)? In formulating our questions, we are allowed several variables: (1) the strength of the individual pulses themselves (e.g., whether 90°, 180°, or other), (2) the number of pulses in a sequence, (3) the time intervals between the pulses themselves (the interpulse interval, designated by the Greek letter *tau*), and (4) the time interval that elapses until the entire pulse sequence is repeated (the repetition time, often abbreviated "TR"). The interpulse interval is usually much shorter than time of repetition. These variables can be adjusted to elicit the desired information. The answers that the body gives to our different questions are in a special "code" contained in the signal from the tissues.

In the next section, we discuss a specific pulse-sequence—the spin-echo—and how the body's response to it contains information about relaxation times.

A COMMON PULSE-SEQUENCE: SPIN-ECHO

Having discussed tissue response to the simplest question—a single pulse of radio-frequency energy—we can explore tissue response to a more complicated question—the spin-echo pulse-sequence. In the simplest form of this pulse-sequence, the tissues are exposed to two pulses: first, a 90° pulse, followed some milliseconds later by a 180° pulse. In this example, the interpulse interval is 15 milliseconds.

As we would expect from the previous experiment, the response to the 90° pulse consists of a free-induction decay signal lasting a few milliseconds. By the time the 180° pulse is applied (15 milliseconds later), the signal is completely gone. As we would expect, the 180° pulse is not itself followed by a strong signal. However, an interesting phenomenon is observed some time after the 180° pulse: the voxel emits a signal that rises from zero to a distinct peak 15 milliseconds after the 180° pulse (and 30 milliseconds after the 90° pulse) (Figure 6–17). Since this peak came at twice the time between the first and second pulses, it is referred to as an *echo*—by analogy to an audible echo. It is actually an echo of the first 90° free-induction decay, made possible by the second (180°) pulse. It

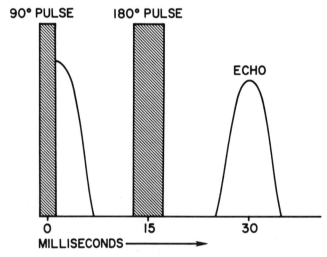

FIG. 6–17. In a typical spin echo pulse sequence, the sample is exposed to a 90° pulse, followed 15 milliseconds later by a 180° pulse. The 90° pulse is followed by free induction decay. Some time after the 180° pulse, a signal is emitted from the tissues, which rises to a peak at 30 milliseconds. The shape of this spin echo is like two 90° free induction decay curves placed back-to-back.

seems to arise spontaneously, since it does not immediately follow a pulse. This separation from the relatively intense excitation pulse is an advantage, electronically, because it allows the very weak return signal to be more clearly distinguished by the receiver.

A person standing on an extended flat surface and clapping his hands once would hear only the single sound directly from his hands. But if there were a large vertical wall 550 feet away, the person would hear, in addition to the actual clap, a second, weaker clap as an echo, about one second later. The sound (traveling at about 1,100 feet per second) arrives at the barrier in one-half second, reverses its direction, and arrives back at its origin another one-half second later. The time of travel to the barrier was half the total time for echo return. The 180° magnetic pulse acts like a magnetic barrier in that it seems to cause an echo at twice the time interval between the 90° and 180° pulses. In MRI, this *time-to-echo* is abbreviated TE.

Origin of Spin-Echo

To understand why the echo is created after the 180° pulse, we need to briefly review why the free-induction decay is so rapid after the 90° pulse.

The loss of the free-induction decay signal is caused by dephasing. To review, in most tissues, T_2 is approximately 30–120 milliseconds, and T_2-star is 5–15 milliseconds, while T_1 is much longer—150–2,000 milliseconds. In the 15 millisecond interpulse interval between the 90° and 180° pulses, very little T_1 decay occurs, but substantial dephasing (due mainly to T_2-star) takes place, and the signal dies nearly completely before the second (180°) pulse. Of the two sources of dephasing, the one that provides tissue characterization is thermal noise from the tissues themselves (T_2). The other (T_2-star) actually causes most of the free-induction decay signal loss, but comes from fixed non-uniformities of the scanner's field. As mentioned previously, the two sources of dephasing are fundamentally different: T_2-star is constant (because it originates from constant non-uniformities) while T_2 fluctuates randomly (because it originates from thermal motion).

To understand the spin-echo phenomenon, consider first the effect of constant non-uniformities at different locations within the voxel under examination. Immediately after the 90° pulse, the phase coherence of all the nuclei in the voxel is high, the magnetization vector lies in the transverse plane rotating at the Larmor frequency, and the free-induction decay signal is maximal. When observed from a rotating frame, the magnetization vector would simply appear to lie stationary in the X-Y plane. Due to T_2-star non-uniformities, the hydrogen nuclei at different locations within the voxel, which were originally locked in phase following the 90° pulse, precess at slightly higher or lower Larmor frequencies, and consequently lose their phase relationship. Because the non-uniformities are constant, the rates of precession of individual nuclei at various points in this field are constant, and the nuclei lose their phase coherence at a predictable rate.

The effect of the 180° pulse is to act as a magnetic barrier, making the nuclei come back into phase at the same rate as they went out of phase. As the nuclei come back into phase, the signals from the individual nuclei are again in phase; and a signal (the echo) is measured.

The reversal of the drifting apart of phase has been compared to a group of race horses that start simultaneously. Several seconds after they leave the starting gate, they occupy various positions along the track, because they are running at different speeds. If their direction were somehow instantaneously reversed, and they continued to run at the same speeds, they would, after a period of time equal to that between the start and the reversal, arrive back at the gate simultaneously. The 90 pulse is analogous to the release from the gate. The 180° pulse corresponds to the unnamed mechanism for causing the horses to change direction; their arrival back at the starting gate is the spin-echo. Because it takes as long to come back into phase (after the 180° pulse) as it took to go out of phase, the time-to-echo is twice the 90°–180° pulse interval.

We can use the magnetization vector (in a rotating frame of reference) to analyze this dephasing and refocusing. After the initial excitation pulse, the magnetization vector would appear to lie stationary in the transverse plane. As the nuclei dephase, the magnetization vector breaks into many smaller vectors, drifting clockwise and counterclockwise at constant rates, like a fan being opened. The

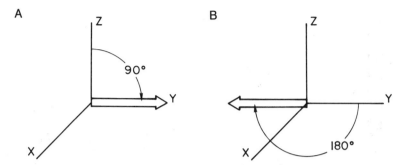

FIG. 6–18. A 90° pulse drives the magnetization vector into the transverse plane (**A**). A 180° pulse applied immediately after the 90° pulse rotates the vector into the opposite side of the transverse plane (**B**). If there is no time interval between the two pulses, they are equivalent to a single 270° pulse and produce a free-induction decay signal. If, instead, a short interval of time is allowed between the 90° and 180° pulses, the phenomenon of spin-echo occurs.

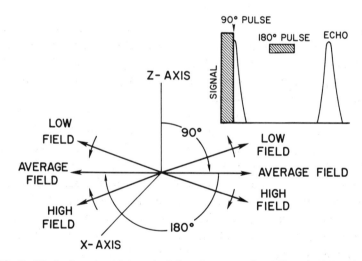

FIG. 6–19. In the short interval of time between the 90° and 180° pulses, some dephasing of nuclei occurs. The direction of phase shift is indicated by the arrows on the vectors fanning out clockwise and counterclockwise in the transverse plane, to the right of the Z-axis. After the 180° pulse, they lie in the opposite side of the transverse plane (to the left of the Z-axis). The arrows on these vectors indicate that the nuclei are coming back into phase. As the nuclei go out of phase (after the 90° pulse) the signal falls off. As they come back into phase (some time after the 180° pulse) the echo signal is produced. The phenomenon of spin-echo occurs because dephasing and rephasing occur at constant rates, due to T_2-star constant non-uniformities of field strength.

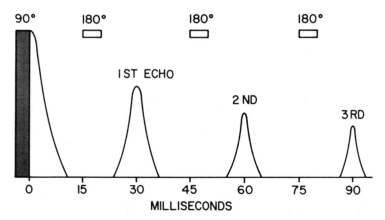

FIG. 6–20. By repeating 180° pulses after the initial 90° pulse, multiple echoes can be generated.

180° pulse causes the dispersing motion of these vectors to reverse. Subsequently, at the time of echo, we would see the many smaller vectors come back together, like a fan being closed. (A more detailed explanation of spin-echo using the magnetization vector is to be found in Figures 6–18 and 6–19.)

The spin-echo produced by the 180° pulse is actually an echo of the free-induction decay produced by the preparative 90° pulse. The echo can be considered a "resurrection" and doubling of the apparently vanished 90° free-induction decay. The echo's shape is determined by the free-induction decay curve's shape. Because the nuclei come into phase at the same rate as they went out of phase, the echo curve is symmetrical: the rising half of the echo curve is the mirror image of the free-induction decay curve. After reaching maximum coherence (the top of the echo curve), the nuclei again go out of phase at approximately the same rate as after the initial 90° pulse, the falling half of the echo curve very closely reproduces the original free-induction decay curve.

It is possible, by repeating several 180° pulses at appropriate intervals, to produce several echoes after the initial 90° pulse. Each new 180° pulse has the effect of reversing the constant dephasing that has occurred since the previous pulse. The ability of pulse sequencing to produce multiple spin-echoes demonstrates the indestructibility of T_2-star dephasing, since echoes can be resurrected several times by subsequent 180° pulses, following a single 90° pulse (Figure 6–20).

From this discussion, we see that the spin-echo is an artifact due to inherent, fixed T_2-star non-uniformity of the MRI scanner's main field, gradient fields, and non-uniformity of tissue magnetic susceptibility. In itself, the echo has nothing to do with tissue T_2. *If, somehow, these constant non-uniformities could be eliminated and the field could be made perfectly uniform, no spin-echo would occur.* Such discussion is purely academic, however, because placement of a patient in the field introduces non-uniformities.

Determining T_2 from Spin-Echo

The constancy of the field non-uniformities throughout the voxel being imaged causes T_2-star dephasing to occur at a constant rate. The effect of the 180° pulse is to cause the nuclei to come back into phase at the same rate as they went out of phase. At the time they come back into phase, the peak of the echo occurs. While the dephasing effects of T_2-star can be reversed by a 180° pulse, those of T_2 cannot, due to their random nature. The echo is thus weaker than the free-induction decay by the amount of T_2 dephasing that has occurred during the time-to-echo.

T_2 represents unpredictable dephasing that "nibbles" away at the spin-echo. *T_2-star creates the echo, T_2 erodes it.* In multiple-echo sequences, the height of successive echoes decreases by T_2. If regional numerical measurements of T_2 are sought, they can be calculated from the rate of erosion between two or more successive echoes from the region (Figure 6–21).

T_2 has a significant effect on the echo because, in most T_2-weighted sequences, the time-to-echo is chosen to span the likely T_2 values of the tissues. Since most healthy soft tissues have a T_2 in the range of 30–100 milliseconds, the time-to-echo is adjusted to fall in the range of 30–120 milliseconds. In clinical MRI, scans usually are constructed from the spin-echo, rather than from the free-induction decay following the 90° pulse. In a common spin-echo sequence, three stimulating pulses are used: the 90° pulse, followed at 15 and 45 milliseconds by 180° pulses, giving rise to two

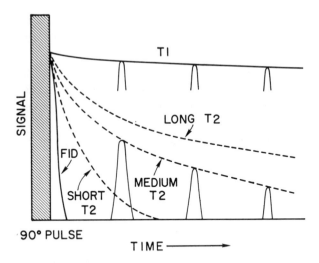

FIG. 6–21. If the only source of dephasing were T_2-star constant non-uniformities of field, the only source of echo degradation would be T_1 (energy loss). This hypothetical case is shown at top by the solid line connecting tips of echoes. But in tissues, repeated echoes decline much more rapidly due to T_2 (random, thermal motion dephasing). *Dashed lines* indicate erosion of multiple echoes in tissues with short, medium, and long T_2.

echoes, at 30 and 60 milliseconds, respectively. In regions of short T_2, rapid degradation of the echo occurs, the signal measured is weaker, and the region appears darker. Conversely, in regions of long T_2, less degradation occurs, the echo signal is stronger, and the region remains bright.

Where there is a region of interest with a long T_2, this can be emphasized by using longer interpulse intervals, to produce later echoes. By the time the later pulses occur, regions of short T_2 have eroded echo signals, and appear dark, while regions of long T_2 have strong echoes and appear bright against the surrounding healthy brain. For example, by delaying the 180° pulses, (e.g. to 45 or 60 milliseconds after the 90° pulse) later spin-echoes (e.g. at 90 or 120 milliseconds) are obtained, and these are useful in detecting regions with pathologically prolonged T_2. By 120 milliseconds, the signal will have disappeared from most healthy tissues, except cerebrospinal fluid (which has a much longer T_2); so the brain itself appears dark. A pathological region of long T_2 could still be producing an echo at this time and appear bright.

Gradient Echoes

It is possible to use gradient magnetic fields in place of 180° radio-frequency pulses to cause the reversal of phasing that produces the echo. A constant gradient in the Z-axis is applied following the 90° pulse. This now dominates other fixed field uniformities to establish the direction of phase drift. At the time a 180° pulse would normally be applied, the polarity of the gradient is reversed, with its strength exactly the same as before reversal. This reversed gradient causes the phase drift of the nuclei to reverse and refocus, thereby creating an echo. An advantage of using gradients to produce echoes is that exposure of the tissue to the substantial amount of radio-frequency energy in the 180° pulses, and its concomitant tissue heating, is greatly reduced.

Deriving T_1 from Spin-Echo

In spin-echo pulse-sequencing, T_2 has a significant effect on the strength of the spin-echo signal because the time-to-echo is adjusted to be comparable to T_2 of most tissues. T_1, on the other hand, had little effect on the spin-echo because the time-to-echo is much longer than T_1. In the examples above, the time-to-echo of the last echo was 120 milliseconds; T_1 of most tissues is in the range of 150–2,000 milliseconds. How is it possible to encode T_1 information into the scan?

Time of Repetition (TR)

In practice, the tissues are not simply exposed to a single spin-echo pulse-sequence consisting of one 90° pulse followed by one or more 180° pulses. Instead, the entire spin-echo pulse-sequence is repeated at intervals of 0.5–5.0 seconds. This interval is called the *time of repetition* (TR). For example, at a repetition time of 0.5 seconds, a 90° pulse is applied to the tissues every 0.5 seconds. Using the same interpulse interval as before, each 90° pulse is followed 15 milliseconds later by a 180° pulse (Figure 6–22). As expected, each 90° pulse is immediately followed by a free-induction decay signal, and 30 milliseconds later by an echo signal. During

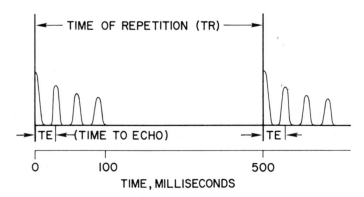

FIG. 6–22. The most common pulse-sequencing used in MRI consists of repeated multiple spin-echo sequences, separated by repetition time, TR. In this example TR is 500 milliseconds. The length of the repetition time affects the amplitude of the next free-induction decay, resulting in T_1 weighting.

these 30 milliseconds, the echo is degraded at a rate T_2. When the repetition time is adjusted to fall in the middle of the range of T_1s of various tissues, the size of the free-induction decay (and thus the spin-echo) in the repeated pulse-sequences is different for different tissues; T_1 information is encoded into the scan and the scan becomes *T_1-weighted*.

To understand why the initial pulse-sequence can affect subsequent pulse-sequences, we need to review T_1 energy loss: A voxel of tissue absorbs a certain amount of energy from a 90° pulse; it loses this energy at rate T_1. This loss of energy is unrelated to the dephasing (from T_2 and T_2-star), which occurs at a much faster rate, and which contributes to the short free-induction decay. The energy loss starts immediately after the initial 90° pulse, and continues long after the last echo, because T_1 is so much larger than T_2 and T_2-star. Although the tissue is "silent" after the last spin-echo signal, this does not mean that the nuclei in the tissue have returned to their equilibrium state; they still possess energy, which they continue to lose.

Dephasing and energy loss can be visualized using the longitudinal and transverse components of the magnetization vector. While the transverse component is dephasing and rephasing, producing the free-induction decay and echo signals, the longitudinal component is growing in the positive Z-direction at the much slower rate T_1. When the transverse component has completely dephased (and shrunk to zero) after the spin-echo, the longitudinal component has regained only a fraction of its original (pre-stimulation) length; it continues to grow upward at rate T_1. If the next repetition of the pulse-sequence is started at a time comparable to the T_1 of a region, its 90° pulse encounters a region of tissue still partially energized (whose longitudinal component has not regained its original length). In this case, the tissue cannot absorb all of the energy that it might from the new 90° pulse, causing the subsequent free-induction decay and its spin-echo in the new pulse-sequence to be correspondingly weaker. On scans constructed from the echo signals of the new pulse-sequence, voxels with a long T_1 appear darker.

In terms of its ability to absorb energy, we can compare a voxel of tissue to a cup being filled with water. A cup can hold only a maximum amount of water—one cupful. When empty, the maximum amount of water can be added to the cup. When partially full, only a portion of a cup of water can be added. In the same way, the hydrogen nuclei in an unstimulated voxel of tissue can absorb only a certain maximum amount of radio-frequency energy—the amount contained in a 180° radio pulse. When the nuclei in a voxel are still partially saturated with energy, the voxel can absorb only a portion of energy from a new 180° pulse.

In our earlier discussion we learned that when voxels in a plane of tissue are exposed to a single 90° pulse, they give free-induction decays of comparable amplitude because of their similar water content. In repeated pulse-sequences, the amount of energy a voxel absorbs from a 90° pulse (and the strength of its free-induction decay) depends on how much energy the voxel has lost since the previous 90° pulse. Because the echo for each voxel is a "resurrection" of its free-induction decay, the heights of the spin-echoes for the voxels also reflects T_1. In general, for a given tissue voxel, the amplitude of its free-induction decay increases with more prolonged repetition time. This occurs because the tissues have had more time to undergo T_1 relaxation and are able to absorb more energy from the new pulse (Figure 6–23).

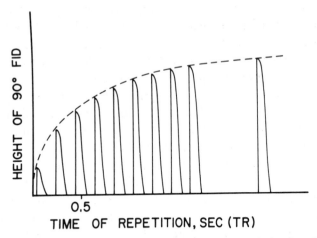

FIG. 6–23. This figure shows the amplitude of the free-induction decay of a repeated pulse sequence, and its relationship to repetition time. At short repetition times, the region has little time to undergo T_1 relaxation and cannot absorb much energy from the next 90° pulse; its free induction decay is correspondingly small. At longer repetition times, the region has more time to undergo T_1 relaxation, absorbs more energy from the pulse, and its free-induction decay is stronger.

Examples of Repetition Times

Using examples of short and long repetition times, we can see how the scans they produce are correspondingly T_1- and T_2-weighted.

T_1 Weighting

The first repetition time to be examined is 0.5 seconds. This repetition time is effective in creating T_1 contrast of tissues, because T_1s of various tissues are scattered above and below 0.5 seconds. At 0.5 seconds after the initial 90° pulse, regions of long T_1 still retain much of their energy, while regions of short T_1 have almost completely relaxed. Because these regions differ in degree of energy retention, they absorb differing amounts of energy from the new 90° pulse. Regions with long T_1 will have decayed less and consequently absorb less energy from the next 90° pulse; the subsequent

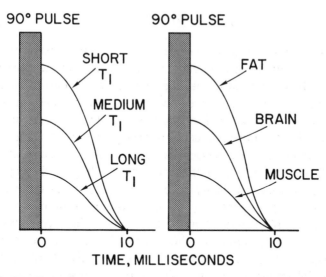

90° PULSE   90° PULSE

SHORT T₁   FAT

MEDIUM T₁   BRAIN

LONG T₁   MUSCLE

0   10   0   10

TIME, MILLISECONDS

FIG. 6–24. The free-induction decays of fat, brain, and muscle at a repetition time of 0.5 seconds. A tissue with a short T_1 (such as fat) will have undergone nearly complete T_1 relaxation; consequently it absorbs more energy, has a large free-induction decay curve, and appears bright. Brain, with a medium-long T_1, undergoes less relaxation and has a smaller free-induction decay curve. Muscle, with its long T_1, undergoes the least relaxation, gives the weakest free-induction decay curve, and appears dark.

free-induction decay and echoes will be correspondingly weaker. Regions with short T_1 have, by 0.5 seconds, lost most of their energy; they absorb more energy from the second 90° pulse, and have a larger free-induction decay (and echo) after the second 90° pulse. On MRI scans reconstructed from echoes of the repeated pulse-sequence, regions of long T_1 appear darker than those of short T_1. Fat, for example, which has a T_1 of about 150 milliseconds, goes through about three T_1s by 0.5 seconds and appears bright on the image. A tissue with a very long T_1, such as cerebrospinal fluid, hardly relaxes at all before the second pulse and appears dark (Figure 6–24).

At a repetition time of about 0.5 seconds, MRI scans are *T₁-weighted*, meaning that the brightness of various tissues depends upon their T_1.

T_2 *Weighting*

If the repetition time is extended to 2.0 seconds, longer than the T_1 of most cellular tissues, enough time elapses for most tissues in the slice being imaged to lose their energy and return to their pre-stimulation state. Each succeeding pulse-sequence encounters tissues that are all essentially in an unstimulated state; T_1 has little effect on the free-induction decay of various tissues or on the echoes of the successive pulse-sequences. Most regions produce, after the new 90° pulse, free-induction decays that are large and comparable in amplitude (because the hydrogen content of various soft tissues is fairly uniform). Apparent T_1 regional differences are minimal, and T_1 does not affect contrast on the final scan. (The exception to this range of T_1 is cerebrospinal fluid, which has a T_1 close to that of pure water [about 2.7 seconds]. At 2.0 seconds, it still retains a substantial amount of energy . When the next pulse-sequence starts, the cerebrospinal fluid absorbs less from the 90° pulse, and appears relatively dark on the image against the brighter cellular tissues.)

With long repetition times, the free-induction decay signals produced by various cellular tissues are all strong and equal, but the efficiency with which the echoes are produced varies from region to region, as a function of regional T_2. Regions of long T_2 appear brighter, while those of short T_2 appear darker. MRI scans made from the spin-echoes of a 2.0 second (or longer) repetition time reflect almost entirely regional T_2, and are therefore said to be T_2-*weighted*.

By using repetition times between 0.5 and 2.0 seconds, MRI scans can present a combination of T_1- and T_2-weighting; the proportion of T_1- vs. T_2-weighting depends on the repetition time.

Using even longer repetition times minimizes regional differences in T_1, thus allowing T_2 to dominate regional image brightness. For example, repetition times of 4–5 seconds and a time-to-echo of perhaps 200 milliseconds produces a bright cerebrospinal fluid with almost no visible soft tissue. The MRI scan produced using this repetition time appears like an old-fashioned myelogram (a radiographic procedure in which iodinated oil replaces spinal fluid). This is an example of how MRI has replaced a painful, traumatic procedure with one that is completely non-traumatic. The physician can use the interpretive skills learned from myelography; there is now rarely a reason for performing myelography.

SOURCES OF REGIONAL IMAGE BRIGHTNESS: A SUMMARY

An MRI scan displays a slice of tissue as regions of varying brightness. Clinical images are usually created using repeated spin-echo pulse-sequences; the image is formed from the echoes. Each scan has on it a line of print stating the repetition time and time-to-echo. The brightness of a region in the image depends upon the strength (amplitude) of its spin-echo signal. To understand regional brightness and its relation to tissue characterization, it may be helpful to summarize the factors determining this echo strength.

There are two factors influencing the amplitude of the spin-echo: (1) the height of the free-induction decay (of which the echo is a resurrection), and (2) the amount of T_2 erosion of echo that occurs between the free-induction decay and its echo.

When the free-induction decay signal is stronger, the echo signal following it is correspondingly stronger. We know that the strength of the free-induction decay signals of successive pulse-sequences is a function of both the region's T_1 and the repetition time, the time separating the repeated pulse-sequences. At long repetition times (of 2.0 seconds or longer), the effect of T_1 on the free-induction decay is minimal, and all voxels in a plane of tissue produce free-induction decays of comparable amplitude. At long repetition times, T_1 contrast is minimized. At shorter repetition times, comparable to the T_1 of tissues, the heights of the free-induction decays of different voxels become differentiated according to their respective T_1. A repetition time of 0.5 seconds tends to emphasize T_1 of soft tissues: the scan is T_1-weighted.

Whatever the height of the free-induction decay, its echo signal is degraded at the rate T_2; some T_2 information is always included in the scan. Scans made with a repetition time of 0.5 seconds, although T_1-weighted, still contain T_2 information. With longer repetition times (of 2.0 seconds, for instance), T_1 information is minimized, leaving the dephasing effects of T_2 as the primary source of differences in echo strength between different regions; the scan is T_2-weighted.

INVERSION-RECOVERY

Another pulse-sequence in common clinical use is the inversion-recovery pulse-sequence. This sequence has the advantage that it can measure T_1 and almost eliminate T_2 effects from the scan. In general, it provides finer anatomical detail and better gray-white matter contrast than T_2-weighted scans.

In inversion-recovery, a 180° pulse is applied to the tissues first, followed by a 90° pulse after an interval of time comparable to T_1 of the tissues (in the following example, 0.5 seconds). The 180° pulse inverts the magnetization vector from the positive Z-axis to the negative Z-axis. Because the magnetization vector is entirely longitudinal, there is no transverse component and no emitted signal. Imme-

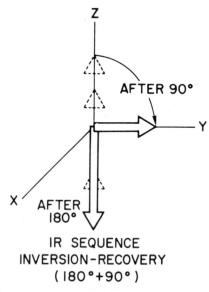

IR SEQUENCE
INVERSION-RECOVERY
(180°+90°)

FIG. 6–25. The inversion-recovery pulse-sequence consists of a 180° pulse followed some time later by a 90° pulse. After the 180° pulse, the longitudinal component grows in the positive Z direction, at rate T_1. The 90° pulse tilts the vector into the transverse plane, providing a readable signal.

diately after excitation, the magnetization vector begins to grow in the positive Z-direction at rate T_1. How much the vector grows in the positive Z-direction during 0.5 seconds is determined by the T_1 of tissue in the voxel but cannot be measured because there is no transverse component, and thus no signal.

To create a measurable transverse component, a 90° pulse is applied to the tissues 0.5 seconds after the 180° pulse. This pulse tips the longitudinal magnetization vector into the transverse plane; a free-induction decay follows the 90° pulse. The strength of this signal is related to the amount of T_1 decay that has occurred since the initial 180° pulse (Figures 6–25 and 6–26). This free-induction decay signal may be measured directly, or, because it is difficult to

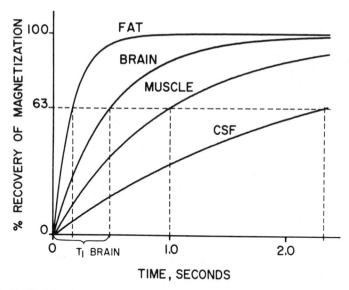

FIG. 6–26. Fat, brain, muscle, and cerebrospinal fluid (CSF) are shown undergoing T_1 relaxation after a 180° pulse. Each tissue is recovering at a different rate: at 0.5 seconds, the three cellular tissues are widely separated in their percentage of recovery; an inversion-recovery scan made at this pulse separation shows considerable contrast between these four tissues. At 2 seconds, the three cellular tissues have nearly completely relaxed; the CSF requires substantially longer. A scan made with this pulse separation shows little contrast among the cellular tissues, but shows strong CSF/cellular tissue contrast.

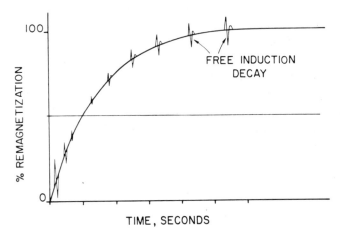

FIG. 6–27. The solid rising curve represents T_1 recovery after the initial 180° pulse. The spikes represent the free-induction decay following the 90° pulse, after the indicated pulse separation. The amplitude of the free-induction decay signal is the same at two different times, after the initial 180° pulse. From a scan made with a specific pulse separation, it is impossible to determine what degree of relaxation the tissue has undergone. (Compare to Figure 6–7.)

measure the re-emitted signal immediately after the intense burst of energy in the 90° pulse, an early echo of the free-induction decay can be produced by applying a 180° pulse soon (perhaps 10 milliseconds) after the 90° pulse, producing an echo (at 20 milliseconds) as in the standard spin-echo sequence. Using the echo in this way to indirectly measure the free-induction decay introduces a slight T_2 effect into the scan.

One problem with the inversion-recovery pulse-sequence is the lack of a simple relationship between T_1 and the amplitude of the free-induction decay signal creating the regional image brightness. Two inversion-recovery sequences, differing only in repetition times, can produce the same strength signal from the same voxel of tissue. This is true over a large range of repetition times (Figure 6–27).

OTHER PULSE-SEQUENCES

The pulse-sequences described in this chapter are the ones most often used in clinical practice. Many others have been developed but cannot be covered here. However, the basic principles are much the same.

Much of the future development of MRI will be the development of new pulse-sequences. Great potential exists in this area, because there are many variables that can be used in designing a pulse-sequence. Some of these were mentioned earlier in this chapter: pulse strength, the number of pulses, and the temporal separation of the pulses. Although not covered in depth here, there are several other possible variables: the intensity, direction, and timing of gradients; and the phase distortion of the signal from different regions of the image. The computer software controlling the execution of the pulse-sequence and the reconstruction of the final image can be regarded as an additional variable contributing to the design of a pulse-sequence. Each of these factors influences, in some way, the signal elicited from the tissues. Each pulse-sequence is a strategy that asks a specific question of the tissues; the answer to each question is encoded in the free-induction decay signal. The signal measured is very complex and must be analyzed by the scanner's computer so that a usable image may be constructed.

The richness of tissue characterization by MRI, compared to the simplicity of CT tissue characterization, suggests the following analogy: CT is to MRI as the game of checkers is to chess. In checkers there are so few rules and possible variations of the game that no elaborate stategies can be developed. Chess has different rules for each of its six different types of pieces; because chess has so many different possible moves, elaborate strategies can be developed. In MRI, we can think of the different pulse-sequences as imaging strategies whose "moves" consist of pulses of different strengths and time intervals between pulses, as well as gradient interactions and computer programming techniques.

7

The MRI Scanner

A clinical MRI scanner superficially resembles a CT scanner: there is a large gantry into which the patient is placed, a control console, a complex of computers, and various other pieces of electronic apparatus. But in most MRI scanners, the gantry is larger than in CT scanners: it is a cylinder about two meters long; its diameter is one-half to one-third its length. This size and shape is important in patient management, because the anatomical region to be examined must occupy the center of this cylindrical volume; consequently, the patient must be fully inside the gantry during scanning.

The dimensions of the gantry are dictated by the size and placement of the several coils needed to generate the magnetic fields used in MRI. The magnetic fields produced are roughly analogous to the earth's magnetic field of our earlier compass analogy. In our discussion of imaging (Chapter 4), we saw how localization is achieved by means of the magnetic gradient (a magnetic field that changes strength gradually between one position in space and another). The resonant Larmor frequency of a hydrogen nucleus depends on its position within this gradient. An analogous magnetic gradient occurs in the earth's field, which could be used to localize a compass needle on the earth's surface.

The magnetic field required for MRI is very strong, but, in order to form the required gradient, it need vary in strength only slightly from one edge of the imaged volume to the other. In MRI, magnetic gradients are produced using the principle of superimposition: when a volume of space is exposed to several different magnetic fields, the resultant field is the sum of the individual fields. The gradient field in MRI scanners consists of weak gradient magnetic fields superimposed on a strong, uniform field (the main field).

The strength of the main field is the most common characteristic used to describe a scanner: current human scanners range in strength from 0.02 to 2.0 tesla. (One tesla is 10,000 gauss.) In addition to being extremely strong, the main field must also be extremely uniform spatially; it must remain constant throughout the scan cycle. Onto the main uniform field are superimposed the weaker, non-uniform gradient fields, which typically increase in strength by about one gauss per centimeter through the region being imaged. This represents a change in main field strength of about 0.25% from one edge of the cross-section to the other. The main field is on continuously throughout the course of an MRI scan, but the gradient fields switch on and off and change intensity many times. The main field and gradient fields are generated by different sets of coils within the scanner gantry. (Permanent magnet scanners do not use coils to generate the main field.) In terms of cost, those producing the main field are most important.

MAIN FIELD MAGNETS

In most clinical MRI scanners now marketed, the main field is generated by *electromagnets*—magnets that use electric current to produce a magnetic field. There are two types of electromagnets employed in MRI scanners: *superconductive* and *resistive*. Another type of magnet—a *permanent* magnet—is marketed by several major companies and shows promise for future development. The type of magnet used is often used to classify the entire MRI scanner: it is either a *resistive, superconductive,* or *permanent magnet* scanner.

It is thought by many people that the strength and uniformity of the main field is of paramount importance in establishing the quality of images produced by a scanner. But with experience it has become clear that there is much more to a scanner than just the strength of the main field. Gradient and antenna coil design, excitation and reception coils, computer software, and scanning strategies (pulse-sequencing) are each critical elements in the system—each is but a link in a chain of quality. This does not diminish the importance of the quality of the main field, but to classify (and evaluate) the entire scanner only on the basis of the main field's strength and the means of generating it, is unjustifiable. At times, the marketing of MRI scanners has resembled the marketing of automobiles in the 1950s and '60s; during those decades, the car with the larger engine was assumed to be better. A similar "horsepower race" has taken place among manufacturers of MRI scanners. In the past, marketing strategies have often focused on the strength of the main magnet; the assumption being made that "stronger is better." In one instance, a manufacturer chose 0.4 tesla for the field strength of their scanner simply because their main competitor manufactured a scanner with a 0.35 tesla field.

Electromagnets

Both resistive and superconductive electromagnets are based on a principle demonstrated by Danish scientist Hans Christian Ørsted early in the nineteenth century: When an electric current flows through a wire, a magnetic field is created in the space around the wire; the strength of this field diminishes as the distance from the wire increases (Figure 7–1). This principle of electromagnetism has been used in many electronic devices, but developing electro-

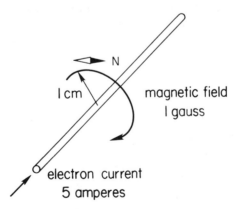

FIG. 7–1. Current passing through a wire creates a magnetic field around the wire. The direction of the field follows the "right hand rule": if one extends the thumb of the right hand in the direction of the current, the four curled fingers represent the direction of the magnetic field, indicated by the direction of the compass. By definition, the strength of the magnetic field one centimeter from a wire carrying 5 amperes of current is one gauss.

magnets capable of creating the large volume of uniform magnetic field required by clinical MRI has been an engineering challenge.

Design of Electromagnets

The details of electromagnet construction (for both superconductive and resistive) vary between designs, but in general, many circular coils encircle the region of the body to be examined. The coils are housed in the gantry of the scanner, each coil being made of many strands of wire or metal foil. The coils are shaped and positioned precisely, and the electron current passing through them is constant. The size of the coils and the geometry of their placement creates an acceptably uniform field throughout the volume of tissue being imaged; the constancy of the electric current ensures the stability of the magnetic field during the time needed for imaging.

To understand why this arrangement of circular coils of an electromagnet can create a uniform field, we can note a theoretical model developed in the nineteenth century: When an infinitely fine wire is spirally wound around the surface of a non-magnetic sphere, and an electric current is passed through the wire, the magnetic field created in the cavity of the sphere is perfectly uniform (Figure 7–2). Such a spherical magnet is not used in MRI scanners, for practical reasons: This design leaves no access holes for the patient; and the creation of access holes would cause the field to bulge out at these

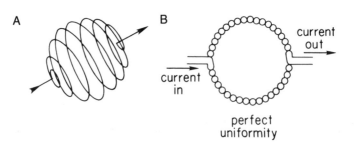

FIG. 7–2. In a theoretical model, current passed through a fine wire wound spirally around an imaginary sphere produces a uniform field within the sphere, shown (**A**) obliquely and (**B**) in midline cross section.

holes, thereby distorting the field. Although not used in practice, knowledge of this theoretical model allows us to understand the designs used in resistive and superconductive systems, both of which achieve uniformity of field by using circular coils of a metal possessing good conductivity.

The major problem to overcome in the design of electromagnets is electrical resistance. At room temperature, every metal exhibits electrical resistance, producing heat when an electric current is passed through it. The manner of dealing with this electrical resistance defines the two types of electromagnets. In resistive MRI scanners, the wire is allowed to stay near room temperature, and the heat produced is physically removed. In superconductive MRI scanners, the wire is cooled to temperatures near absolute zero, at which temperature the metal loses its resistance; and the electric current flows without producing heat.

Resistive Scanners: Geometry of Coil Arrangement

In resistive scanners, four coils are used to produce the main magnetic field. They are parallel to one another and the outer two

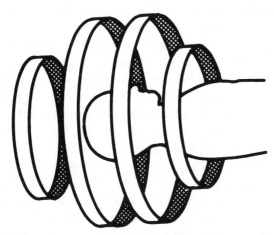

FIG. 7–3. In resistive scanners, four separate coils of a size and position that approximate a sphere are used. This permits patient access, while providing acceptable uniformity in a sufficiently large volume.

are smaller in diameter than the inner two, so that the four coils approximate the surface of a sphere, like parallels of latitude on a globe. Although this design does not produce perfect uniformity in the entire volume contained by the coils, it does create acceptable uniformity in a volume large enough to be useful for imaging and at the same time provide patient access (Figure 7–3).

The four-coil arrangement only approximates the surface of a sphere; the coils do not conform exactly to it: The end coils are made somewhat smaller. This design creates a slightly higher field near the apertures, thus tending to repel the bulging magnetic field back inside, and to compensate for the defect in magnetic field produced by the patient access holes.

Heat Production in Resistive Scanners

In resistive scanners the coils are made of either foil or wire of a highly conductive metal, such as copper or aluminum. Although aluminum and copper are good conductors of electrons, these metals do offer measurable resistance and, consequently, produce significant amounts of heat.

The use of these metals in resistive magnet coils limits field strength to about 1,500 gauss (0.15 tesla). This practical limitation is due to the heat dissipated in the coils by the very large electric currents required. To create a 1,500 gauss field requires 200–250 amperes of electric current that, in an MRI resistive coil system, generates about 50 kilowatts of heat. To double the field strength would require doubling the electric current, which, unfortunately, results in quadrupling the heat dissipation. To raise the field strength to 3,000 gauss would require dissipating 200 kilowatts of heat. Fifty kilowatts of heat is manageable, but 200 kilowatts of heat would be difficult to dissipate in a hospital setting. Heat from the aluminum foil is dissipated by passing distilled water past each coil assembly and then sending the heated water to an external heat exchanger. Fifty kilowatts of heat is approximately the amount produced by a passenger automobile engine; the heat exchanger is equivalent to an automobile's radiator.

A further problem in generating a magnetic field using resistive magnets is the production of a strong continuous electric current.

Any fluctuation in the electric current results in a corresponding fluctuation of the magnetic field and consequent loss of image quality. Fortunately, modern power supplies are capable of regulating the current to within one part per million and are available at a reasonable cost. The magnetic field produced is correspondingly constant with time.

Field Uniformity in Resistives

Field uniformity is poorer with resistive magnets than with superconductive magnets for several reasons. First, the volume of uniformity is smaller. In general, the larger the magnet relative to the patient, the greater will be the volume of acceptable uniformity. In resistive magnets, the coils are made small to reduce the amount of aluminum used in an attempt to minimize heat production. This small coil size constricts the size of the volume of acceptably high uniformity. No resistive coils are perfectly shaped, nor can they be perfectly spaced. Positioning of the coils is a particular problem in the presence of the main magnetic field. When the current is switched on, and the main field produced, the field produces magnetomotive forces that tend to pull the coils toward their common center. This makes it difficult to position the coils, and to maintain them exactly parallel and undistorted.

As with superconductive systems, ferromagnetic materials (structural steel, etc.) in the external environment of the magnet further distort the external field, and thus the field within the magnet. Shimming can be used to finely tune the magnet and counteract such distortion. To this end, movable steel rods can be positioned outside the coils. In resistive systems, threaded adjustments are often provided to position the coils.

The electronic current supply is very stable but, inevitably, imperfectly regulated. As a consequence, the magnetic field necessarily fluctuates slightly.

Advantages of Resistive Magnets

Despite their limited field strength, resistive main coils have some attractive features: manufacturing cost is low compared to superconductive coils; electrical power cost is only $6–$10 per hour while operating; and they can easily be turned off when not in use. Resistive scanners produce good clinical images, even at the low field strengths of most resistive systems (0.02–0.2 tesla). Resistive scanners cannot, however, meet the field strength and uniformity requirements for some applications, such as chemical-shift spectroscopy.

Superconductive Magnets

The electrical resistance of most metals is roughly proportional to their absolute temperature (measured in degrees kelvin). Put simply: cooling causes their electrical resistance to drop. (For example, the resistance of a tungsten filament in an incandescent light bulb is about ten times greater when it is lit than when it is unlit.) As they are cooled from higher temperatures to temperatures near absolute zero, most metals show a drop in resistance that is nearly linear. With many metals, however, at a specific critical temperature a few degrees above absolute zero, the resistance falls abruptly to zero

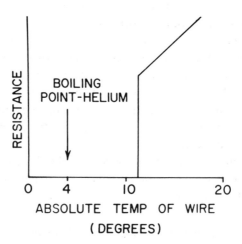

FIG. 7–4. When cooled, most metals show a drop in electrical resistance. Some show a complete loss of resistance (superconductivity) near absolute zero.

(Figure 7–4); their conductivity becomes infinite, and they are said to be superconductive. An electric current started in a superconductive wire circulates indefinitely. The exact temperature at which superconductivity occurs varies from metal to metal and from alloy to alloy. Ordinary lead (Pb), for instance, becomes superconductive below 7.4° kelvin. In MRI it is desirable to use conducting metals or alloys whose critical temperatures are as high as possible. The niobium-titanium alloys used in MRI scanners become superconductive at temperatures in the range of 10–20° kelvin. The coils are cooled by liquid helium, which boils at 4.2° kelvin.

At installation, the coils of the MRI scanner are cooled, the current is started, and, when the desired field strength is reached, a superconductive link is closed. Thereafter, no further power is required. For practical purposes, the current runs indefinitely (so long as adequate cooling is maintained); the drop in field strength is no more than a few gauss each year. Because the flow of electric current is constant, the magnetic field created within the MRI scanner is constant; it is essentially a powerful permanent magnet.

In 1987, a new class of ceramic superconductors was announced. They can become superconducting at temperatures greater than 100° kelvin, allowing cooling with only liquid nitrogen. If these materials can be commercially fabricated into dependable wires, much less expensive MRI superconductive magnets may be possible.

Coil Configuration

In the resistive magnets discussed above, the size of the coils is minimized in order to reduce the amount of conducting metal used and to reduce heat production. Because there is no electrical resistance in superconductive magnets, no heat is produced: there is no longer a critical constraint on the length of wire used and the size of the coil. A superconductive coil consists of many small superconducting wires; the total length of wire in a coil can be eleven to two hundred kilometers, depending on the manufacturer. Superconductive coils with diameters as large as two meters have been manufactured. Because the coils can be made larger relative to the patient, the volume of tissue being imaged also increases; the degree of field uniformity within this volume also improves.

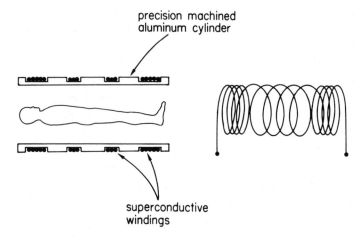

precision machined
aluminum cylinder

superconductive
windings

FIG. 7–5. In superconductive MRI scanners, the coils are positioned in grooves on the outside of a precision-machined cylinder of aluminum. Acceptable field uniformity is obtained by using more turns of wire near the ends of the cylinder.

In resistive magnets, we saw how four coils conforming to the surface of a sphere were used to create a uniform magnetic field. In superconductive magnets, the coils are placed in grooves on the outer surface of a precision-machined cylinder (usually made of aluminum). As a result, all the superconducting coils have the same diameter. The coils are clustered in groups of four or six, with the higher number near the ends of the cylinder. Although the coils have the same diameter, placing more of them at the ends of the cylinder than near the center creates a stronger magnetic field at the ends. This minimizes bulging of the field at the openings, creating a volume of uniform magnetic field within the cylinder. The effect is comparable to the theoretical model of the sphere wrapped with wire (Figure 7–5).

The cylinder and its coils are suspended in liquid helium (4° kelvin). The helium container is suspended in a vacuum chamber that in turn is surrounded by liquid nitrogen (70° kelvin) . This is surrounded by another vacuum chamber. This rather elaborate assembly is understandably expensive to manufacture, and it requires considerable expertise in order to make a reliable product. At present, about six companies make essentially all of the clinical superconductive magnets.

Liquid Gas

Liquid nitrogen is readily available, but liquid helium is not. The cost of the latter is therefore variable. Helium is present underground in natural gas deposits, as a result of alpha decay of long-lived radioactive substances such as thorium and its daughters. Because it is a noble monatomic gas and has an atomic mass of only four, helium has a low boiling point, making it easily isolated from natural gas by liquefaction. Since helium cannot burn, it is a useless component of natural gas. Although easily produced by anyone having a substantial supply of natural gas, there has not been widespread recovery of helium (and particularly its liquefaction) because of the lack of a commercial market. Helium is much less expensive in the United States than elsewhere because of a governmental stockpiling of critical elements.

Preventing helium boil-off from an MRI scanner is a formidable problem that can best be appreciated by thinking of the outside room as an oven 300 degrees (celsius) hotter than the liquid helium inside the scanner. Typically, loss of helium from early superconductive magnets was about 500 milliliters per hour, vented to the outside atmosphere. At the 1990 liquid helium price of about $5 dollars per liter, annual helium cost was $15,000–$20,000. Added to this is the cost of liquid nitrogen. Although a greater volume of nitrogen than of helium boils off, it is much less expensive. If helium loss is considered a serious economic problem, closed refrigeration systems are available to re-liquify the helium. Such a refrigerant system can be located at some distance from the scanner; it consumes 5–20 kilowatts of power. Modern superconducting systems boil off only about 150 milliliters per hour, with a corresponding reduction in cost.

Superconductive magnets are permanent magnets in the sense that, once the current in them is started, the magnet maintains the field without outside power. Other than replenishing their liquid gases and maintaining the vacuum, they should require no major maintenance for several years.

Quench

Superconductivity is a delicate phenomenon that can disappear seemingly without reason. When this happens, the magnet is said to *quench* and the field drops to zero. Fear has been expressed in the past lest a quench occur with a patient in place. Quenches are most likely to happen while technicians are working on the system, and a patient is unlikely to be inside during these times. With the advanced design of modern superconductive magnets, a quench is unlikely to be dangerous to a patient in the magnet or a person nearby, because it takes several seconds for the field strength to fall to zero. In a recent experiment, an anesthetized human-sized pig was subjected to the quench of a 1.7 tesla field. In this experiment, the field collapsed over a period of about twenty seconds, with no evident harm to the animal. In an ordinary quench, the superconductive wire remains nearly intact physically and, as the field collapses, the considerable energy stored in the field is largely dissipated in the coil, heating it and boiling off some or all of the helium. In the unlikely event of a mechanical disaster (a major earthquake, for instance) that splits the gantry open, breaking the coils and spilling much liquid gas, the rapidly collapsing field could cause electrical arcing at unpredictable places, but the major threat to life probably would be asphyxiation from the large volumes of inert gases released.

After a total quench, depending on its cause, down time can be several hours to several weeks. First, the cause must be determined; it is usually some defect in the liquid helium containment. When the problem has been corrected, a substantial fraction (perhaps all) of the 300–500 liters of the helium content of the magnet will probably have to be replaced. After cooling, the build-up of field typically requires several hours. Quenching of superconductive magnets might be thought of as the MRI equivalent of X-ray tube failure in CT; both are expensive sources of unreliability. Fortunately, quenching is much rarer than X-ray tube failure, but usually each quench is more costly.

Field Strength of Superconductive Magnets

These large, stable magnets offer high field strength and great uniformity of field over an extended period of time. It might be thought that a zero resistance conductor could carry an infinitely large current, but there is a practical limit on the current any given conducting metal can carry at a given temperature and field strength. Above this limit, the conductor becomes resistive, causing heating and then quenching. It is entirely practical to make a 2–4 tesla clinical magnet and, indeed, some currently installed scanners have 2 tesla magnets, although they may also be run at lower strengths. There are also several 4 tesla MRI scanners in operation. Whether such strong fields will find wide clinical use is still controversial. One capability of high field scanners is chemical shift spectroscopy. As discussed in Chapter 6, a stronger main field in the MRI scanner results in a longer magnetization vector and stronger NMR signal from the tissues. This extra signal is required to perform chemical shift spectroscopy.

Many of the currently available superconductive systems use fields of about 0.35–0.6 tesla, often well below their rated maximum. This seems entirely adequate for high-resolution clinical hydrogen imaging.

Federal regulations require that public access to all building space having magnetic field strength of more than 5 gauss must be controlled. Higher field magnets require correspondingly larger controlled space. This extensive field outside the gantry, the fringe field, is an inherent disadvantage of superconductive electromagnets.

Permanent Magnets

The main magnetic field can also be generated by large permanent magnets. The most common magnets in everyday experience, such as compass needles and bar magnets, are examples of permanent magnets. This type of magnetism is based on the property of ferromagnetism possessed by certain elements (such as iron), alloys, and ceramic substances. These solids have an electronic structure such that, when they are placed in a strong external magnetic field, their atoms align with it, and remain more or less aligned, even after the external field is removed. To some degree, the entire solid remains permanently magnetic. The field of this permanent magnet is constant, with no need for a continuous power supply. No heat is generated, and no liquid gases are needed for cooling. Many everyday electromagnetic devices that require a strong, constant and inexpensive magnetic field use a permanent magnet to generate this field. Examples of such devices are loudspeakers, galvanometer movements, and small electric motors (Figure 7–6).

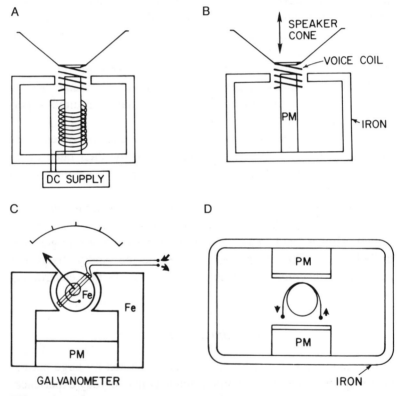

FIG. 7–6. Most modern electronic devices (such as loudspeakers and galvanometers) that require a strong, constant magnetic field use permanent magnets (PM). Before the development of alnico permanent magnets, the strong constant field in a loudspeaker was created by more expensive resistive magnets (**A**). Figure (**D**) shows a simplified MRI permanent magnet with the excitation coil in place.

Although permanent magnets are capable of producing magnetic fields of strengths comparable to those of resistive magnet systems, it is difficult to design a permanent magnet that will produce a field with sufficiently high uniformity over a large enough volume for MRI. Permanent magnet designs have used two magnetic surfaces (pole faces) separated by a gap large enough for a patient. But simply using two flat pole faces does not produce a magnetic field with high enough uniformity. Since magnetic field lines repel each other (much as do electrical charges), they tend to bulge out of any gap in the iron magnetic path, unless they are confined by another design feature. Most permanent magnet designs constrict the bulging of the field in order to achieve the desired uniformity, either by shaping the surface of the pole faces or by using weak electromagnets to "shim" the final field.

Fringe Field in Permanent Magnets and Electromagnets

Two of the major differences between permanent magnets and electromagnets are in the orientation of the magnetic field through the body and in the amount of fringe field produced by each. In electromagnet (resistive and superconductive) systems, the magnetic field passes longitudinally through the body. Within the imaged volume, the field is uniform: The lines of force are parallel. At the gantry openings, the field spreads out into the room, curving out around the scanner and into the opposite opening, forming a complete magnetic circuit. The portion of the magnetic field that extends outside the scanner into the surrounding environment is the *fringe field*, which exists because the magnetic field requires a return path to form a complete circuit. In most electromagnets, this return path is entirely through air. A steel object in the return path distorts the field inside as well as outside the scanner (Figure 7–7).

In permanent magnets, on the other hand, the magnetic field moves directly between the two pole faces, passing transversely through the patient. The pole faces are mounted on opposite sides of a large rectangular or oval steel frame. The magnetic field goes through the air between the pole faces, through the back of one pole face, through the steel frame, and into the back of the other pole

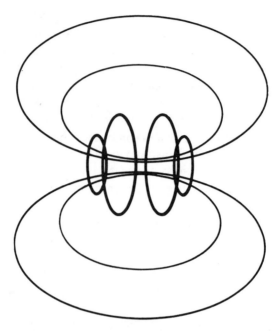

FIG. 7–7. In electromagnets, the field spreads out at the gantry openings, forming a return path through the surrounding air and creating fringe field.

face. Because the return path is almost entirely through the steel frame of the scanner itself, MRI scanners using permanent magnets to generate the main field have very little fringe field. Building modifications due to fringe field pose little problem with permanent magnets (Figure 7–8).

One MRI scanner using a permanent magnet was produced (Fonar Corp.). It had a field strength of 0.3 tesla. Although this particular design was very heavy (90,000 kilograms), it made excellent images and required very little power. It required no liquid gases and could not quench. The initial cost was about the same as superconductive scanners, but it had a negligible maintenance cost and, because of its low fringe field, could be installed in a relatively small (but well-supported) space, with few of the building modifications necessary for MRI scanners using electromagnets. Significantly, this permanent magnet proved that there are no insurmountable engineering obstacles presented by the proximity (and

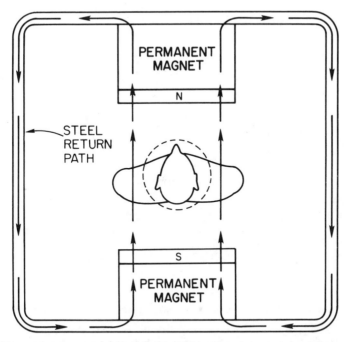

FIG. 7–8. Design of a permanent magnet MRI scanner. Blocks of magnetic material are mounted on opposite sides of a square steel frame. The field passes between the two pole faces and forms a return path through the frame; there is no fringe field. The *dashed circle* represents the region of high field uniformity, acceptable for imaging.

thus interaction) of the gradient coils and other coil units with the nearby pole faces of the permanent magnet. It is to be hoped that there will be further development of permanent magnets—particularly smaller, lighter, and less expensive magnets—to provide the main field. If lighter permanent magnets (3,000–5,000 kilograms) were to become available, an MRI system using this design would have several major advantages: ease of manufacture, low cost, long life without appreciable field loss, low fringe field, minimal maintenance, and only minor building modifications. Such a scanner is now being marketed by Toshiba-America. This system is named "Access" to draw attention to the easy access to patients during scanning. The scanner crudely resembles a four poster bed, with four heavy cylinders of iron making the magnetic return path. An-

MAGNETIZATION

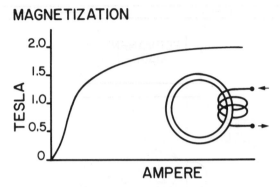

FIG. 7–9. Current passed through a loop of wire wrapped around a circular piece of iron creates a magnetic field, magnetizing the iron. As current load is increased, the iron becomes more magnetized. But between one and two tesla, the iron becomes saturated and cannot be further magnetized. In practice, permanent magnet MRI scanners are limited to about 0.2 tesla field strength.

other manufacturer, Hitachi, has also marketed a permanent magnet scanner having a field strength of 0.2 tesla. This scanner is not too heavy to be impractical; the company has used new, exotic permanent magnet materials that are stronger than traditional materials.

In general, when compared to superconductive magnets, permanent magnets have the disadvantage that their practical field strength is limited to about 0.2 tesla, even if there were no restriction on weight. Permanent magnets have iron in their magnetic circuits, which begins to saturate above this field strength. Increasing the amount of iron in the return path does not entirely avoid this problem (Figure 7–9). Electromagnets can generate much stronger fields because their magnetic return path is through air, which does not saturate. In addition to being unable to achieve the strong field offered by air-path superconductive magnets, it is unlikely that any permanent magnet design will produce the high uniformity required for clinical spectroscopy.

It is possible that MRI scanners using permanent magnets will become common clinical instruments for many applications other than clinical chemical shift spectroscopy, in which very high field uniformity and strength are essential. This situation could be compared to the current role of permanent magnets in laboratory chemical shift (NMR) spectral analyzers (a common instrument in physics and chemistry laboratories). Several companies manufacture such analyzers, each offering a line of analyzers through a range of quality. At the lower (least expensive) end of each line are usually permanent magnet devices. Unexpectedly high uniformity can be achieved because the sampled volume is so small (less than one cubic centimeter).

What Magnetic Field Strength Is Required for MRI?

This has been a highly controversial subject, the center of heated discussion since 1983 when marketing of scanners began in earnest. Generally, each manufacturer promotes its own design, and particularly the field strength of its main magnet, as best. The debate is usually conducted in terms of *low-field* versus *high-field* MRI scanners. Low-field is usually defined as less than about 0.5 tesla, and high-field as greater than 1 tesla. In general, because the costs and limitations of main magnet production increase as the field strength increases, the ideal field is the lowest that will perform the tasks required. Since the tasks MRI will be asked to perform have not yet been fully defined, it is impossible to suggest an ideal field strength. What follows is a general discussion of the advantages and disadvantages of high-field strengths.

Advantages of High Field Strength

Signal-to-Noise Ratio

At higher field strengths, hydrogen nuclei tend to align more (the magnetization vectors for tissue voxels are larger). Consequently, the tissues absorb more energy, and the signal emitted from the tissues is correspondingly stronger. This extra signal can be used for more rapid imaging or for other data manipulation. The fact that the signal strength increases with field strength is of particular importance because there is also a constant background noise emitted from the tissues: thermal motion in the tissues produces a radio signal of its own, consisting of a wide range of frequencies. The amplitude of this background noise is independent of the strength of the magnetic field applied to the tissues. When the strength of the main field is increased, the signal from the hydrogen being imaged increases proportionately, while the background thermal noise remains the same. In the terminology of electronics, the *signal-to-noise* ratio increases.

To use an everyday analogy, when we listen to a distant radio station, the radio receiver automatically increases its sensitivity in order to detect the weak signal. But, in addition to being more sensitive to the desired signal, the receiver also becomes more sensitive to electrical noise. The distant station's signal is difficult to hear because it is mixed with random clicks and hisses—the background electromagnetic noise—that come from many different sources. When we listen to a strong radio station, the receiver's sensitivity automatically decreases, and the background noise becomes less noticeable. The stronger radio station has a better signal-to-noise ratio.

Chemical Shift Spectroscopy

Stronger fields are also important in hydrogen or phosphorus chemical-shift spectroscopy. The nuclei of atoms in an organic molecule are surrounded by clouds of moving electrons. These moving electrons create their own magnetic field, which cancels, to a very slight degree, the field strength to which a nucleus is exposed. In a sense, the surrounding electrons shield the nuclei from the external magnetic field. For nuclei that are magnetic, this slightly lower field strength causes a lowering of the Larmor frequency. This is called *chemical shift*.

The configuration of the cloud of electrons around each nucleus in a particular organic molecule is unique. As a result, each nucleus experiences a slightly different degree of shielding of the external field. When the same magnetic nucleus (of hydrogen or phosphorus, for instance) occurs at several locations in an organic molecule, it possesses slightly differing Larmor frequencies, depending on its location. NMR spectroscopy measures the signal from organic molecules and distinguishes the magnetic nuclei at different locations by their Larmor frequencies. These slightly differing Larmor frequencies are displayed as peaks on a spectrum, each peak corresponding to the position of one magnetic nucleus in the molecule's electron cloud. Each type of organic molecule has a characteristic spectra. Organic molecules can be identified, and distinguished from other types of organic molecules, based on their spectra.

At lower field strengths, it is difficult to use NMR analyzers or MRI scanners to separate spectral peaks of the nuclei. Because the degree of shielding (and corresponding change in Larmor frequency) of any nucleus is small, the Larmor frequencies of nuclei are close, and the peaks of the spectrum are poorly separated. At higher field strengths, not only is the signal from any particular peak stronger, but the resonant frequency of the nuclei increases in proportion to the field strength: spectral peaks are more spread apart in absolute numbers of cycles per second. This simplifies their electronic separation.

The Importance of Mobility in Signal Production

Nuclei of ^{13}C, ^{19}F, and ^{31}P produce very feeble signals that can be measured in living tissues only by chemical shift spectroscopy. To produce sharp spectral peaks a tissue component of possible interest must be freely mobile and unattached to either membranes or large molecules. As a consequence, relatively few substances are identifiable—much less measured—in tissues. (One of the reasons hydrogen nuclei are successfully imaged is that, in addition to emitting a strong signal, they are freely mobile in tissue water.) The lack of mobility of nuclei such as ^{13}C, ^{19}F, and ^{31}P is one reason why chemical shift spectroscopy probably will find few applications in a clinical setting.

Disadvantages of a Strong Magnetic Field

In general, cost rises with field strength. It is probably impractical to create a resistive magnet stronger than about 0.2 tesla, because of heat dissipation problems. To produce stronger fields, the more expensive superconductive magnets must be used. Because of the fringe field created by electromagnets, the amount of building space dedicated to the scanner rises with field strength; as field strength increases, the acceptable 5 gauss field line moves farther away from the scanner, and site preparation costs rise accordingly. For high-field superconductive magnets, the cost of site preparation can be as much as for the scanner itself. The fringe field can be an inconvenience, because it distorts television and computer screen images at considerable distances; many older video cameras cannot be used within 5–10 meters of a magnet.

Elongated ferromagnetic materials in the body (such as some vascular clips) undergo a torque that tends to orient them parallel to the main field of the scanner. The torque is proportional to field strength. Fortunately, most metallic prosthetic materials implanted surgically are not significantly ferromagnetic. Effects on cardiac pacemakers can be expected to be greater at high fields. Pacemaker problems must eventually be solved by redesigning pacemakers if widespread use of MRI is to be implemented.

Higher field strengths result in greater signal strength but also require stronger gradients and, especially, stronger excitation pulses, causing tissue heating. In high-field machines, typical transmitter power (during a pulse) is about 10 kilowatts, comparable to many commerical radio broadcast transmitters. Although all commercial scanners meet conservative governmental requirements for power deposition, it should be noted that in multiple-echo pulse-sequences the transmitter is on much of the time. These pulse-sequences require the body to be exposed to a series of strong (180°) radio pulses, each of which may be 1–8 milliseconds long and repeated 20–50 times per second. This can result in considerable tissue heating. In modern spin-echo imaging, this problem is greatly minimized by using repeated reversal of the Z-gradient field—rather than transmission of 180° inverting pulses—to produce the echoes. The power transmitted into the tissue, and consequent tissue heating, is thereby greatly reduced.

Another problem that increases with higher field strength is noise heard by the patient during scanning. The strong electrical currents intermittently present in the various gradient coils cause them to act like the voice-coil in a loudspeaker: each time the electric current switches on or off, the position of the coil changes abruptly and a click or thump is heard by the patient. With multi-slice excitation, the gradients must be changed many times per second, making a very loud machine-gun-like noise that is disturbing to many patients. This gradient coil noise increases with field strength and un-doubtedly contributes to the claustrophobic response in some pa-tients.

In a quench, the energy stored in the field must be dissipated; during a quench, this energy rises with the square of field strength. Any ill effects of a quench on patients or the apparatus itself would increase accordingly.

In electromagnets (superconductive and resistive), the spread of the fringe field must be taken into account. In permanent magnets, the return path is within the scanner itself, but in resistive and super-conductive scanners, it spreads out to include surrounding space. Fortunately, in the first 5–10 meters, the field strength falls off with the inverse cube of distance, rather than inverse square. This means that the field strength falls by a factor of eight rather than four each time the distance from the magnet is doubled.

Where the field converges at the openings of the magnet, large gradients exist. These draw nearby ferromagnetic materials, such as wrenches and gas tanks, into the ends of the gantry. This phenome-non, known as the *missile effect*, is more pronounced at higher field strengths.

In conclusion, one should not judge a scanner solely by the type of magnet used to generate its main field, the field strength, or the uniformity. Most of the currently available superconductive systems use fields of about 0.35–0.5 tesla, considerably below their theo-retical capability. This appears sufficient for high resolution clinical imaging. One resistive scanner, with a field of only 0.02 tesla is now being marketed by Instrumentarium of Helsinki. Its ability to produce clinically useful images invites re-evaluaton of the entire question of field strength. If such low-field resistive scanners enjoy continued success, the development of MRI scanners based on small permanent magnets might also be stimulated.

Field Uniformity

When discussing field uniformity, it is important to consider both the uniformity of the magnetic field and the volume over which the uniformity exists. In standard chemical analytic spectrometers (the major practical application since Purcell and Bloch published their discovery of NMR in 1946), the required uniformity is extremely high—less than one part in ten billion—but the volume is extremely small—about five millimeters in diameter. Such extreme uniformity is unnecessary in clinical MRI scanners. The most stringent requirements for MRI scanning are in chemical shift spectroscopy, which requires about one part in ten million uniformity over a three-to-five centimeter cube. For clinical hydrogen imaging, the requirements are much less strict. Depending upon spatial resolution requirements and the image reconstruction method used, uniformity of one part in ten thousand over a volume fifty centimeters in diameter may be adequate.

As the imaged volume is reduced, any given magnet shows greater field uniformity. (In a larger volume more imperfections are likely to be encountered.) Although a scanner's field may have a uniformity of one part in a hundred thousand over a 50 centimeter volume (and thus be unacceptable for chemical shift spectroscopy), a small surface (topical) coil might examine a volume only 5–8 centimeters in diameter. Within this sub-region of the total field, the uniformity would be higher and possibly acceptable for spectroscopy.

It might be thought that improving field uniformity in MRI scanners would be a good means of obtaining better image resolution in clinical hydrogen imaging. In fact, there is little reason to be preoccupied with extremely high uniformity to improve image resolution. In ideal circumstances, clinical MRI seems to be limited to spatial resolution of about 0.5 millimeters, since there is approximately this much movement in the most cooperative patient, due to heart and respiratory movements.

GRADIENT COILS

Whether the main magnet is superconductive, resistive, or permanent, it generates throughout the course of the scan a constant magnetic field of the required strength and uniformity in a volume large enough to be clinically useful. In order to image tissues, slight gradients must be created. These gradients are generated by adding to or subtracting from the main field in a controlled and systematic manner. These non-uniformities are created by *gradient coils*

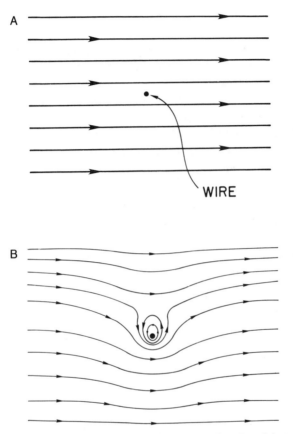

FIG. 7–10. A: Parallel lines of force represent uniformity of the main field. There is no current flowing in the wire, so it does not affect the main field. **B:** A wire carrying current out of the page generates a surrounding magnetic field that interacts with the main field. According to the right hand rule, the field of the wire opposes (and cancels) the main field above the wire but reinforces the main field below the wire.

housed in the gantry of the scanner. The gradient coils are themselves electromagnets, which generate a magnetic field when current is passed through them. Because the gradient fields are so much weaker than the main field, much less power is needed to create them, and heating is not a problem. Because the gradients are switched on and off many times during the course of a scan, current flows intermittently. To understand how the MRI scanner uses gradient coils to create magnetic gradients, we might first examine how current in a single wire interacts with the main field.

Electric current moving through a wire produces a circular magnetic field, expressed graphically as concentric lines. The direction of the magnetic field is determined by the direction of the current, using the right-hand rule. The direction of the field is reversed by changing the direction of the current (Figure 7–10).

A current-carrying wire placed perpendicularly to the main field distorts the field. On one side of the wire, the direction of the wire's own field is the same as the main field: there the fields reinforce, and the strength of the total field on that side of the wire is increased. On the other side of the wire, the direction of the wire's field opposes the main field: the fields cancel, and the total field on that side of the wire is decreased (Figure 7–10A + B). The function of the gradient coils is to use these additions and subtractions in order to modify the main field, so that its strength changes in a continuous fashion in the desired direction. The coils are circular or semi-circular loops of wire. There are three separate sets of gradient

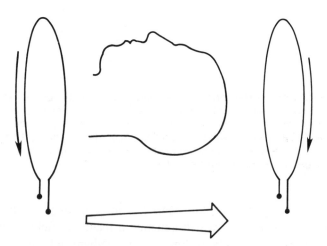

FIG. 7–11. The longitudinal Z-axis gradient is created by two circular coils of wire. Current is passed in opposite directions through the two coils, as shown. The main field is reinforced near the coil on the right and diminished near the coil on the left, resulting in a magnetic gradient between the two coils.

coils; each set produces a gradient along one of the coordinate axes: X, Y, and Z.

Z-axis Gradient

The longitudinal Z-axis gradient is the most easily understood. It is produced by two circular loops of wire positioned perpendicularly to the Z-axis, on either side of the region to be examined (Figure 7–11). To produce the gradient, current is passed in opposite directions in the two loops, clockwise in one and counterclockwise in the other. The field produced by one coil adds to the main field near that coil; the field produced by the other coil subtracts from the main field near it. Between the two loops, across the region being imaged, the resulting main field shows a gradual transition from a slightly higher field strength at the adding coil, to a slightly lower field strength at the subtracting coil. This forms the Z-axis gradient.

X and Y Gradients

The Z-axis coils described above are easily positioned in the gantry, because they are circular and conform to the cylindrical patient opening. Such pairs of circular coils cannot be used to create gradients along the X and Y axes, because circular coils positioned along the X and Y axes would not conveniently fit the shape of the gantry. Instead of circular coils, semi-circular coils are used. These half-loops are paired, one half-loop on each side of the gantry. Current is passed in opposite directions in these two half-loops. The magnetic field produced in one half-loop adds to the main field near that loop; the field produced by the other half-loop subtracts from the main field near it. The result is a gradient between the two half-loops, in the transverse plane across the patient.

For example, to create an X-axis gradient, the two pairs of half-circles are arranged on the left and right of the patient, as shown in Figure 7–12. When current is passed in opposite directions in these two half-loops, as shown, the field from the half-loop on the right subtracts from the main field on the right, and the field from the other half-loop adds to the main field on the left, creating a gradient in the transverse plane across the patient, along the X-axis, with

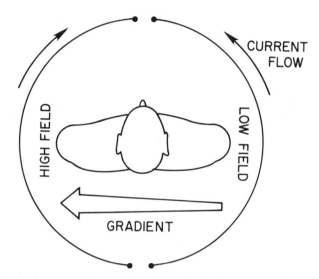

FIG. 7–12. A transverse gradient is created using opposed semi-circular loops of wire in which current flows in opposite directions. The field from one semi-circular loop adds to the main field, and the field from the other subtracts from it, forming a gradient. Here, the arrangement for X-axis gradient coils is shown. If the main field has its north pole at the patient's feet and its south at the head, the gradient coils will add to the main field on the left and subtract from it on the right, according to the right-hand rule.

field strength increasing from right to left. Another pair of half-loops in the gantry above and below the patient similarly create the Y gradient.

In practice, two pairs of half-circles, on opposite sides of the patient, are used to create a transverse gradient across the volume of tissue being imaged. In an MRI scanner, each of these opposed half-loops is paired and connected by wire running in the Z direction. The straight connecting wires produce no magnetic field component in the Z direction and so do not add to or subtract from the main field. Only the curved portions—the half-loops in the X-Y plane— are active in creating X and Y gradients. The pairs of curved half-circles and the wires connecting them are called *saddle coils*, because of their shape (Figure 7–13). The X- and Y-axis saddle coils,

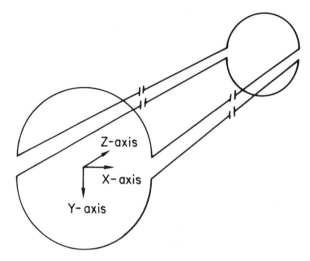

FIG. 7–13. MRI scanners use saddle (Golay) coils to produce the transverse gradients (here the arrangement for the Y gradient is shown). Each saddle coil consists of two semi-circular loops of wire connected by straight wires. The semi-circular portions are active in creating the gradient; the straight portions serve only to connect the loops and do not contribute.

and the circular Z-axis coils, are oriented as shown in Figure 7–14. When currents are passed through them in the directions shown, the desired gradients are created.

In the absence of a Z-gradient, X- and Y-axis gradients add to form a single gradient in the X-Y plane. By adjusting the relative strengths and polarity (up-or-down, left-or-right) of the individual X and Y gradients, a single gradient of any strength and direction in the X-Y plane can be produced—the vector sum of the X- and Y-gradients.

In Chapter 4, we described the original (and simplest) means of imaging a transverse slice of tissue. First, isolation of this slice of tissue is achieved by applying a Z-axis (longitudinal) gradient to the body and exposing the tissues to a pulse of radio-frequency energy of a single wavelength. After the slice has been excited and thus isolated, the Z-axis gradient is turned off. Further localization is obtained by applying a second gradient, this time in the transverse

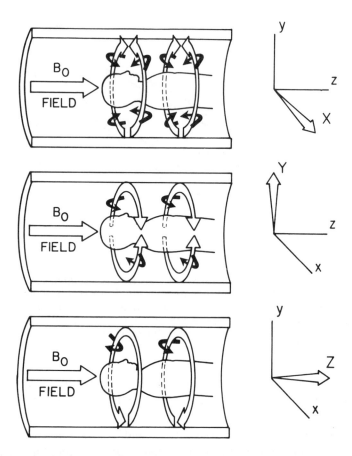

FIG. 7–14. *White arrows* show the direction of current in the X, Y, and Z axis gradient coils; *black arrows* represent the field produced by coils. These fields interact with the main field (B_o), resulting in the gradient along the coordinate axis shown on right.

X-Y plane. The transverse gradient localizes the hydrogen nuclei along a set of parallel lines, perpendicular to the vector representing the gradient (see Figures 4–4 to 4–10). The direction of this transverse gradient is determined by the strength and polarity of the individual X and Y gradients: by appropriate changes in the strength and polarity of the individual X and Y gradients, the direction of the net X-Y gradient can be rotated progressively like the hands of a clock.

Each successive rotation of the gradient localizes the nuclei along a new set of parallel lines.

Spatial Orientation of Imaged Plane

Although this sequence of gradients (first Z and then X-Y) is used to image a transverse plane, other anatomical planes (sagittal, coronal, etc.) can be imaged with equal facility, by exchanging roles between X, Y, and Z gradients. Since the gradients are controlled electronically, there are no moving parts involved in changing the orientation of the imaged plane, or indeed anywhere in the MRI process. This ease of changing orientation of slice selection is a major advantage over X-ray CT, in which scans are limited to within a few degrees of transverse.

The precision of these gradients must be as good as modern engineering allows. The coils must be physically shaped and positioned with great care and must remain stationary during the entire scanning procedure. The amplifiers supplying their currents must provide exactly the right amount of extremely constant current and be able to change from one current level to another and become stable at the new level within about 1 millisecond. Although the controlling voltages, which involve very small currents, are easy to produce with the required accuracy, the amplifiers required to provide the very large gradient coil currents at low voltage require a high level of engineering skill.

EXCITATION AND RECEIVING COILS

In order to stimulate the hydrogen nuclei during imaging, the tissues must be exposed to energy in the form of a radio signal. The signal subsequently emitted from the tissues must also be detected. These functions are carried out by *transmitting* and *receiving coils* contained in a separate unit wrapped closely around the region of the body being imaged.

As discussed in the Appendix, to be most effective, the radio signal must enter the tissue at right angles to the main field. Since the main field in most scanners is longitudinal, the signal must enter the tissues transversely (in the X-Y plane). A simple wrap-around circular transmitting coil would be ineffective, because it would produce only a longitudinal signal. Instead, a saddle coil is used to produce the transverse signal. In design it is similar to the saddle coils used to produce the transverse X- and Y-axis gradients.*

Because they must be held in precise position, the gradient coils are usually housed in the gantry separate from the patient compartment. They define the spatial coordinates in the patient. The excitation and antenna coils are placed around the patient and are removable. Both body and head coils are commercially available, the latter being smaller. It is possible to make one coil serve as both the excitation and receiving antenna, since excitation and detection are not carried out at the same time. With the growing interest in surface coils, which are smaller antenna coils placed directly on various parts of the body, it has become convenient to use separate coils for excitation and receiving: the ordinary larger antenna coils (such as for body or brain) can be removed and the surface coil used instead.

SURFACE COILS

Much of the future of magnetic imaging lies in the ability to image small tissue volumes at high resolution. This is accomplished by means of surface receiving antenna coils, called simply *surface coils*, made of circular copper wire or tubing placed on the surface of the body, over the region to be examined. They can be designed to lie flat, or configured to fit the shape of some anatomical region, such as the knee.

A simple circular surface coil defines an approximately spherical

---

*Saddle-shaped transmitting and receiving coils are used in most commercial scanners because the main field is longitudinal (along the Z-axis). In permanent magnets and at least one experimental resistive unit, the main field is directed transversely (perpendicularly) to the body. In such transverse main fields, simple circular coils—rather than saddle coils—are most efficient for excitation and reception. Such coils generate a longitudinal radio signal, perpendicular to the transverse main field, providing the most efficient excitation. Similarly, they produce the most efficient reception. Below 1 tesla, such a simple coil will produce about twice the signal of a comparable saddle coil. Above this field strength, the relationship between orientation of antenna and field direction becomes less important.

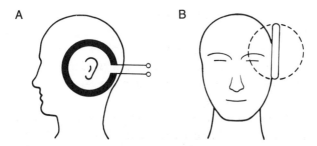

FIG. 7–15. A: A surface coil is a small receiving antenna consisting of a circular loop of copper wire or tubing, placed on the surface of the body. **B:** It detects signal in a spherical volume, but because one hemisphere contains only air, all of the signal comes from the hemisphere of tissue.

volume of space, with the coil itself at the equator of the volume. The coil usually is only a receiving antenna, sensitive to signal emitted from tissues within this volume. With the coil in place on the surface of the body, the hemisphere away from the body contains only air and produces no signal. All of the signal comes from the other hemisphere, the one containing the tissue to be imaged (Figure 7–15).

Except for the substitution of the surface receiving coil for the full-body receiving coil, the scanning apparatus remains the same. Full-body excitation coils are used, and the procedure for imaging an entire slice of tissue is followed. But instead of the signal being received from the entire slice, the surface coil detects a signal from only that portion of the excited slice lying within the small hemispherical volume. This is then processed by the computer as though it were the signal from an entire slice.

There are three major advantages of surface coils. First, a small anatomical region is spread over the entire display matrix, thereby improving spatial resolution; resolution is improved by a factor of at least two, compared to scans of an entire slice. This is particularly important in small structures such as the orbit. Second, the close proximity of the surface coil to the tissue being imaged results in a high sensitivity to signal from this small volume. Third, because the surface coil receives signal from only a small volume, there is less thermal noise mixed with the desired image signal: signal-to-noise ratio and image quality are improved. (The surface coil receives signal from only a portion of the slice being imaged and random thermal noise from only the small amount of tissue in the hemispherical volume. In contrast, a saddle-coil used to image an entire slice of tissue receives noise from a much larger volume of tissue, compared to the slice being imaged.)

Although technically much more complex, MRI is, in almost all clinical circumstances, more useful than X-ray CT. We anticipate that during the next decade, virtually all medical diagnostic X-ray procedures will be replaced by procedures performed by less expensive, faster, and more compact MRI scanners.

8

Sample MRI Scans

The MRI scans in this chapter are courtesy of Jeffrey Phillips, M.D. and George Bartzokis, M.D.

A

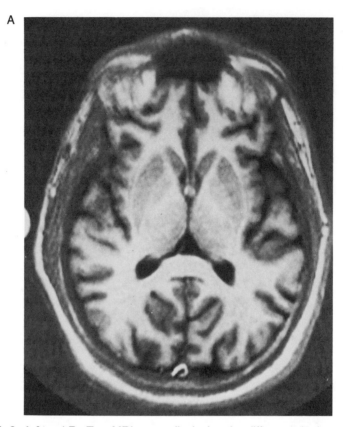

FIG. 8–1 A and **B.** Two MRI scans displaying the difference in tissue contrast obtained by using two different pulse sequences. On the left is a T_1-weighted sequence. On the right is a T_2-weighted sequence. The dark linear structures are rapidly moving blood in veins and arteries. On the T_1-weighted scan, the gray matter and white matter are much better differentiated and the cerebrospinal fluid appears dark. Conversely, on the T_2-weighted scan, the cerebrospinal fluid appears bright. (See Chapter 6 for discussion of T_1- and T_2-weighting.)

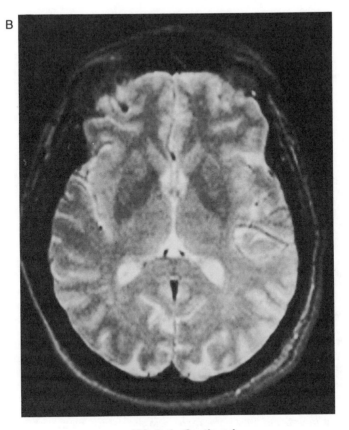

FIG. 8–1. *Continued*

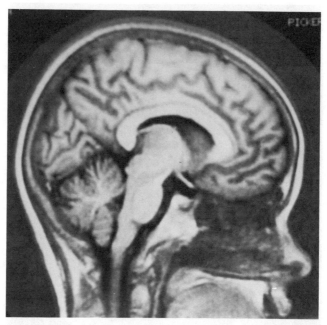

FIG. 8–2. A sagittal section directly through the midline of the head. The nose and upper lip give orientation. As one enters any point on the outer surface of the head, there is a light gray line that represents the outer layers of the scalp, and then a bright line, which is fatty tissue in the deeper layer of the scalp. Proceeding toward the center of the head, there is then a dark line representing compact bone of the skull. Then a bright layer of the skull that represents fatty bone marrow in the central portion of the skull. Continuing inward, there is a dark layer, representing the compact bone of the inner layer of the skull. The cerebral gyrii are well shown, and the large curved structure in middle of the head is the corpus callosum, which contains about 100 million nerve cell fibers and connects the two cerebral hemispheres. Many other anatomical structures can be seen at the base of the brain.

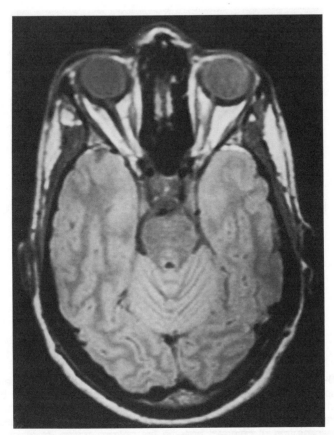

FIG. 8–3. A transverse section through the head showing the eyeballs and optic nerves. Several of the muscles that rotate the eye are also visible in the orbit as gray structures against the bright fat, which fills most of the space of the orbit. In the very middle of the head is the pons, and the dark area near its lower border is the aqueduct of sylvius, in which there is surging cerebrospinal fluid. It appears dark because it moves at right angles to the plane of the section. Below the aqueduct of sylvius, and running obliquely to the right and left of it in a "V" pattern, are several alternating light and dark bands. These bands represent the folds of the midline cerebellar cortex.

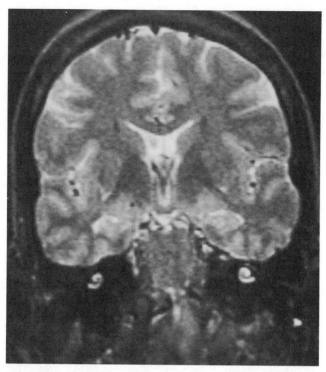

FIG. 8–4. A coronal view of the brain through the middle of the cerebral hemispheres. This picture is of special interest because of the two bright, curved structures lying beneath the brain. These are the cochlea—the sensory microphones for hearing. They stand out as bright objects against the dark background of compact bone in the petrous region. In all of these pictures, if the region is dark, it means that it is either bone, gas, or rapidly moving fluid (blood or cerebrospinal fluid).

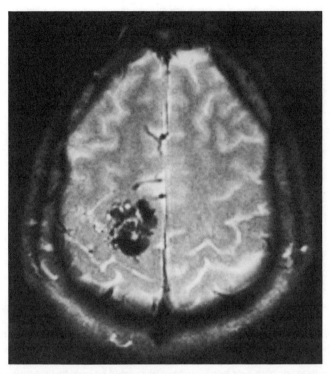

FIG. 8–5. A transverse section near the top of the cerebral hemispheres. The dark object in one hemisphere is an arterio-venous malformation, a collection of abnormal blood vessels in which the arteries are connected directly to veins and a large blood flow is present. The other vessels at some distance from the main mass are veins or arteries that have enlarged to carry the large amount of blood that the tumor requires.

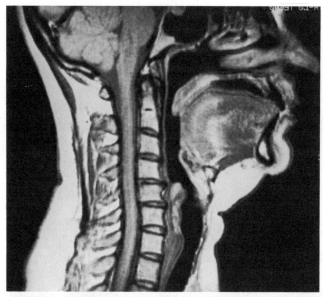

FIG. 8–6. A sagittal midline T_1-weighted scan of the neck in a normal patient. The spinal cord can be seen passing downward in the spinal canal. The vertebral bodies can be seen as bright, rectangular objects in front of the spinal canal. The vertebrae appear bright on a T_1-weighted scan because bone marrow is fatty and, consequently, has a short T_1. Other than the thin layer of compact bone surrounding most bones, the bone is largely filled with the bright-appearing bone marrow.

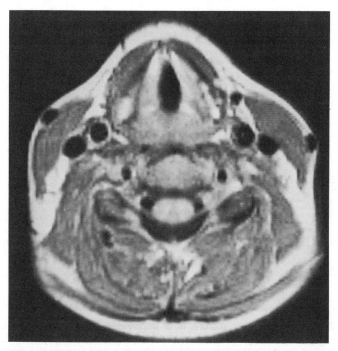

FIG. 8–7. A transverse section through the neck at the level of the larynx. The dark areas here are filled with either air, rapidly moving blood, or moving cerebrospinal fluid. The oval dark area near the top in the midline is the air path in the larynx. Below and to the left and right are paired vessels appearing to be of about the same diameter; the one nearest the larynx is the common carotid artery and the dark area lateral to that is the internal jugular vein. Below and toward the center of the section are the vertebral arteries. The spinal cord is plainly seen as are two of the nerve roots leaving the spinal cord and passing out into the nerves of the arm and hand.

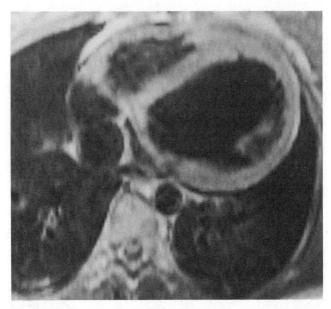

FIG. 8–8. This complex picture is a transverse view, low in the chest, showing the two large cavities in the heart (the ventricles). The larger, thick-walled cavity is the left ventricle. Above it and toward the midline is the right ventricle. The dark circle below the thick-walled left ventricle is the descending aorta.

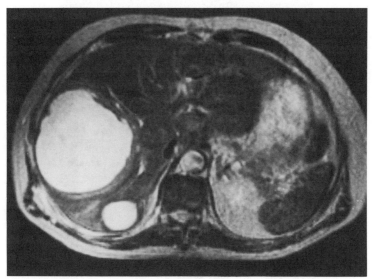

FIG. 8–9. Transverse section through the upper abdomen, showing liver, spleen, and a very large, bright, sharply demarcated tumor in the liver.

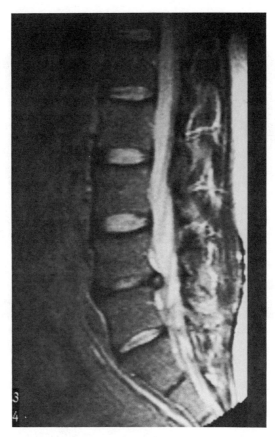

FIG. 8–10. Midline sagittal section of the lower lumbar spine and the spinal canal. The bulging object protruding into the spinal canal is a herniated intervertebral disk. Each of the rectangular bodies is one of the lumbar vertebrae. Between the vertebral bodies are the intervertebral disks, which appear bright. As one progresses downward, the lowest intervertebral disk is seen between the fifth lumbar vertebra and the first sacral vertebra. The vertebrae making up the sacrum, progressing out of the picture downward and to the right, are fused together and thus do not have intervertebral disks. The spinal cord ends at about the upper-most intervertebral disk on this photograph; the nerves that go out between the lower vertebrae all pass downward from the spinal cord and emerge from the spinal canal near intervertebral disks. These disks have a relatively fluid center and a firmer outer shell. Occasionally, under excessive pressure and in the presence of degeneration of the disk, the disk herniates—some of the fluid contents create a "blister" that protrudes out into the canal. Most of the symptoms of herniated disk are caused by the consequent pinching of the nerve, which passes nearby through an opening that allows it to distribute to external structures. Before MRI, these herniated disks could be seen only by injecting an opaque oil dye, and then X-raying the spine. This procedure, myelography, was painful and has now fallen largely into disuse.

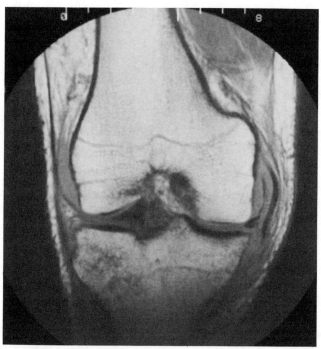

FIG. 8–11. Transverse section of a knee. The upper bone is the femur, and the lower bone is the tibia. The slippery space between is the knee joint. Again, the interior of both of these bones is bright because they are largely fatty bone marrow, while there is a dark rim of compact bone surrounding the marrow. This compact bone has water in it, but the water is in a crystalline form, has an exceedingly short T_2, and for practical purposes produces no signal. Compact bone therefore appears black on MRI scans. The kneecap, or patella, is not in this section, but would cover roughly most of the center of the joint.

9

Advantages and Limitations of MRI

MRI sections superficially resemble those made by CT (at least in the transverse plane) because both create black-and-white cross-sectional images of the body. As can be seen from the MRI scans presented in the previous chapter, there are many differences between the images the two modalities produce. It would be a mistake to consider MRI as just the next generation CT scanner. The differences between the two types of scans, and the advantages and limitations of each technique, come from the nature of the probes they use, and the hardware needed to produce them. In CT, the probe used is a narrow beam of X-rays. In MRI, the probe consists of magnetic fields used in conjunction with radio energy. Due to the nature of the magnetic probe used in MRI, this technique possesses several fundamental advantages: (1) tissue can be characterized in a number of ways, (2) any plane in any orientation can be imaged, (3) bone is invisible, so all anatomic regions can be examined, (4) no contrast medium is required, and (5) there is no ionizing radiation.

At the present time, there are also several disadvantages: (1) the complexity and high cost, (2) the long scan time, (3) the noise and isolation experienced by patients during scan, and (4) the exclusion of a substantial fraction of patients due to pacemakers, metallic artifacts, and inability to cooperate. The first two of these—complexity and long scan time—are the subject of active research and development, and improvement can be expected. However, the last two—gradient coil noise and the exclusion of many patients—are more fundamental problems whose solutions are not yet apparent.

ADVANTAGES OF MRI

Invisibility of Bone in MRI

In conventional radiography and CT, bone is prominently displayed because X-rays interact strongly with bone. Bone appears bright in CT scans and imaging of certain anatomical regions, such as the base of the brain and the spinal cord, is limited. But bone does not interact with the magnetic fields and radio signals used in MRI. Compact bone is essentially invisible. One consequence of this is that fatty bone marrow (which is invisible to CT) can be seen; indeed, it is the only bone structure visible by MRI.

In Chapter 4, we learned that MRI involves several steps: (1) creation of carefully controlled magnetic fields in the region to be imaged, (2) exposure of tissue to pulses of radio waves, (3) detection of the signal subsequently emitted from the tissues, and (4) processing of this signal by a computer to reconstruct the final image. Bone interferes with none of these steps. Bone has low magnetic susceptibility, so it does not appreciably distort the magnetic fields created by the scanner; soft tissues experience the same magnetic field regardless of the density or shape of adjacent bone. Because bone does not interact with radio waves, neither the strong radio signal transmitted into the body nor the radio signal subsequently re-emitted from the soft tissues is affected. The signal detected by the MRI scanner's antenna is thus unaffected by the presence of bone.

Bone produces almost no signal of its own. The signal from which the scan is made comes largely from the hydrogen nuclei of water molecules in soft tissues. Soft tissues have a very high water content, and, because much of the water is in liquid form, it is mobile and can be imaged. The signal from compact bone is much weaker, for several reasons. First, the water content of compact bone is only about 25% (by volume)—a fraction of that found in most soft tissues. Another reason is that, while water in soft tissues is relatively mobile, most of the water in bone is probably bound into the bony crystalline structure as water of hydration and so behaves as a solid, having a very short T_2 (less than one millisecond). With this short T_2, the nuclei are completely dephased within ordinary times-to-echo of 20–40 milliseconds. This, together with the low water content, appears to be the major reason for lack of any readable signal from bone. Virtually all of the received signal in MRI is, then, from soft tissues.

When interpreting MRI scans, the loss of the usual radiographic bony landmarks is at first disorienting, but it soon becomes evident that this is a great advantage. Even structures embedded in bone (such as the pituitary, inner ear, spinal canal, or posterior fossa contents) can be clearly visualized. The absence of bone in the MRI scan offers the first opportunity to study all of the bone marrow. Since essentially all bones contain marrow, a postmortem anatomical study of all marrow would be tedious in the extreme and probably has never been done. One of the possible fundamental contributions of MRI could be comprehensive studies of marrow in all of the bones, to seek out possible regional abnormalities.

Ability to Scan Any Plane

MRI can directly scan any plane desired. CT requires physical movement of the X-ray source about the patient, thus restricting imaging to transverse sections. In MRI, the gradient magnetic fields that define the orientation of the plane being imaged are changed electronically, with no moving parts, so any plane through the body can be studied. The fact that MRI scans can be made in various planes with no loss in quality is an enormous advantage in clinical interpretation.

Tissue Characterization: T_1, T_2, and Fluid Movement

The most important advantage of MRI is its ability to provide tissue characterization beyond simple hydrogen distribution. By changing the pulse-sequencing used and the computer software, several tissue characteristics can be explored. The major tissue characteristics currently being exploited are water hydrogen distribution, T_1, T_2, fluid movement (particularly of blood), and magnetic tissue susceptibility.

T_1 and T_2

In Chapter 5, we introduced the principles of tissue characterization. There are two aspects of the behavior of the hydrogen nucleus that can easily be measured by MRI. These are the *time constants*, or *relaxation times*, T_1 and T_2. In the compass analogy, we stated that the time constant T_1 indicates the rate at which energy is lost from the stimulated nuclei, and T_2 indicates the rate at which dephasing of the oscillatory motion of the nuclei takes place. These nuclear properties are not in themselves of interest, but they are strongly influenced by the molecular environment of the hydrogen nuclei and can be used as means of characterizing tissues.

The T_1 and T_2 of pure water, at ordinary field strengths, are both about 2.7 seconds. In tissues, both are shorter, with T_2 being very much shorter than T_1: Tissue T_1 is about 150–2,000 milliseconds, while tissue T_2 is about 20–120 milliseconds. The reasons for the shorter relaxation times of tissue relative to pure water and of differences in tissue relaxation times between different tissues are not clear, but some generalizations can be made. The water in tissue cells has a much greater micro-viscosity than pure water because it is exposed to many macromolecules and membranous surfaces; these serve to slow down thermal motion of water molecules and thus to accelerate T_1 relaxation. In addition, there are many trace paramagnetic substances, such as dissolved gaseous oxygen, that shorten both T_1 and T_2. Elaboration of these relationships between cellular function, structure, and relaxation times is the subject of intensive study and will undoubtedly become considerably clarified.

Most modern scans present a mixture of T_1 and T_2; the degree to which a scan is *weighted* toward T_1 or T_2 is dependent on the exact pulse-sequence used, that is, on the strength of the individual pulses and the timing between them. The direction, steepness, and duration of the gradient fields used during the scan is another variable. T_1-emphasized scans, which often use the inversion-recovery sequence, show excellent gray/white matter differentiation and high spatial resolution. When T_1 of a region is long, T_2 of that region is usually long also. Usually, T_2-weighted images better demonstrate pathological brain lesions.

The relationship of relaxation times to image brightness can be confusing. On T_1-weighted scans, regions of short T_1 usually appear bright, while those of long T_1 appear dark. Body fat, for example, has a short T_1 and appears bright on T_1-weighted scans. Its rapid T_1 relaxation prepares it to absorb a great deal of energy from the next excitation pulse. Consequently, its signal is strong and its image is bright immediately after this next excitation. The shortening of tissue T_1 by paramagnetic contrast agents causes a brighter image for the same reason. On the other hand, regions of long T_1, such as cerebrospinal fluid, retain their energy longer and so cannot absorb as much energy from the next excitation pulse and appear darker on T_1-weighted scans.

On T_2-weighted scans, regions of short T_2 appear dark, and those of long T_2, bright. One advantage of a T_2-weighted scan is that it presents lesions of long T_2 as bright spots on a dark background. In any black and white picture, an object of interest is more striking when displayed as a bright object on a darker background, than as a dark object on a lighter background. Many lesions (for example, cerebral metastases, brain edema, and multiple sclerosis lesions) have a longer T_2 than adjacent healthy brain. On the T_2-weighted scan, the multiple cerebral white matter lesions of multiple sclerosis appear as bright spots in the surrounding darker white matter. T_1-weighted images, on the other hand, usually show these lesions as less obvious dark spots on a field of grayish-appearing white matter. Whichever weighting is used, MRI shows multiple sclerosis lesions with a much greater sensitivity than does CT.

Much experience is required to interpret scans made with various pulse sequences, because so many apparently different images can be made of the same scan slice, using different pulse sequences. The resulting images may look as though they were tissue slices stained by entirely different histological techniques. In practice, it is best to become familiar with a few pulse-sequences and use them instead of trying to tailor each scan to the patient. (A detailed discussion of pulse-sequencing was presented in Chapter 6.)

Even *in vitro* relaxation measurements are not as accurate as one might expect; they are influenced by several obvious variables, such as temperature and oxygen content. Other sources of variability are difficult to pinpoint; estimates of relaxation times from MRI scanners seem to show a wide range for the same tissue in different patients, and even in the same patient upon repeated scans. While gross changes in relaxation times aid in visual interpretation of scans, it would be very useful if accurate and reproducible numbers could also be attached to various regions of the scan. At present, attempts to do so have been disappointing. The literature on this subject has been summarized by P. A. Bottomley (1985).

Imaging of Moving Blood

The entire MRI process presupposes that the nuclei being imaged will be in the same location throughout the sequence of excitation and subsequent re-emission of energy. But blood is moving at a surprisingly rapid rate: in the ascending aorta, as it leaves the heart, its velocity approaches one-half meter per second. The arteries branch repeatedly; on average their total cross-sectional area increases by about 25% at each branching, and the velocity of blood slows accordingly. By the time it has reached a capillary, blood is moving about one millimeter per second; in major arteries in the brain, its velocity is perhaps 10 centimeters per second. This means that even during the brief interval between pulses, the blood travels a substantial distance. It no longer responds to pulse-sequences as does the adjacent, stationary tissue: the moving blood appears black (Figure 9–1).

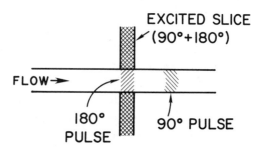

FIG. 9–1. Blood moving rapidly, perpendicular to the plane of excitation, is not in the plane for both pulses of a pulse sequence. Since the same hydrogen nuclei must experience both pulses to produce an echo and be imaged, moving blood produces very little signal (and so appears black).

There are several reasons why blood appears black: (1) If moving nearly perpendicularly to the section being imaged, the same blood may move out of the plane being imaged, and may not receive both the 90° and 180° pulses required for the spin-echo. (2) If moving substantially parallel to the plane of section, the blood will have moved into a new region of both the main and gradient fields, with new field strengths; the spin-echo process will be largely curtailed, since the 180° pulse inversion requires a constant field non-uniformity to allow refocusing of the echo. (3) Blood flowing in a vessel moves faster in the center than it does near the walls. This results in a continuous slippage of layers of blood between the center of the stream and the wall. The velocity profile is approximately parabolic (Figure 9–2). Although this blood is subject to the same thermal motion as stationary tissues, there is a superimposed rotation of water molecules caused by their laminar flow, which further accelerates dephasing. (4) Turbulent flow (such as in narrowed vessels), with its multiple vortices and changes in direction, is still another source of dephasing (Figure 9–3). The latter three sources of dephasing are random and contribute to what is essentially a very short

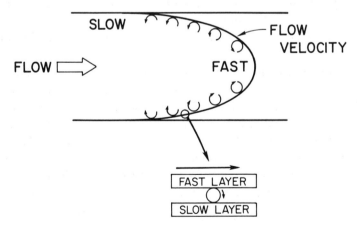

FIG. 9–2. Blood moves faster near the center of the vessel than near the wall. Small arrows show slippage of layers of blood between the center of the vessel and wall. This laminar blood flow further contributes to the lack of signal from moving blood.

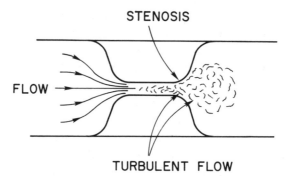

FIG. 9–3. Turbulent blood flow causes increased tumbling beyond that due to smooth laminar flow.

T_2. Moving blood creates a *flow-void*, a regional lack of signal that appears black on the MRI scan.

In the cerebrospinal fluid cisterns at the base of the brain and in the aqueduct of Sylvius, between the third and fourth ventricles, there are substantial tidal movements due to changes in brain volume due to cardiac action and to changes in central venous pressure. These movements of the cerebrospinal fluid are sufficiently fast that they can be imaged; they may become a useful diagnostic aid in space-occupying lesions in the posterior fossa, since these masses could interfere with normal tidal movements. These movements cause some regions of the cerebrospinal fluid to appear darker than others.

To summarize, there are currently four clinically useful tissue characteristics that MRI can define: (1) regional hydrogen concentration, (2) regional T_1 behavior, (3) regional T_2 behavior, and (4) regional rate of bulk hydrogen movement (from one location to another). Undoubtedly, other influences on hydrogen magnetic behavior in tissues will be measured in the future. It is reasonable to expect that most—or perhaps all—invasive arteriography will eventually be supplanted by non-invasive MRI visualization of vessels.

Contrast Media

There is so much tissue characterization already available from a modern MRI scan that it is only rarely that one would wish to introduce a contrast material in order to obtain further information, particularly if there were some danger of toxicity. The most widely researched contrast media are paramagnetic substances. Paramagnetic substances are atoms that are magnetic due to the structure of their outer electron shells, rather than of their nucleus. (One such atom can have the magnetic strength of a thousand hydrogen nuclei.) In even trace tissue concentrations (a few parts per million), paramagnetic substances shorten T_2 enough to be useful as contrast agents. (For a discussion of paramagnetism, see Chapter 5.)

Gaseous oxygen (O_2) dissolved in tissue water is strongly paramagnetic; the chemistry of this is poorly understood. O_2 is promising since it can be administered by inhalation for short periods of time, with no concern for its toxicity. Inhalation of 100% O_2 causes slightly more oxygen to be dissolved in blood, bringing about a slightly shorter T_1 and T_2 in most regions of the body. This could be useful in detecting areas of reduced blood-flow if clinical measurements of T_2 become accurate enough to allow these slight changes to be seen.

Some of the transitional metals such as iron, copper, manganese, and gadolinium are strongly paramagnetic, usually in their oxidized (Fe^{+++}, Cu^{+++}, Mn^{+++}) state, and can be chelated with ethylenediamine tetraacetate (EDTA) or diethylenetriamine pentaacetic acid (DTPA) to allow rapid renal clearance. In brain MRI, these chelates behave much like the iodinated agents in CT because, being polar molecules, they achieve substantial concentrations in brain only in blood vessels and in tissues in which the blood-brain barrier is defective. Although the paramagnetic agents studied to date seem to be non-toxic, rare idiosyncratic reactions may occur. Whenever there is an intravenous injection, there is the remote possibility that, due to human error, some unintended harmful substance might be injected by mistake.

It should be remembered that CT contrast agents were called into use in the very early development of CT, at a time when the resolution of CT scans was very poor; the use of contrast agents helped make the lesions more obvious. There is already so much tissue characterization and high resolution anatomical detail available with MRI without injecting anything that there is not the pressure to develop artificial enhancement agents as there was with CT. Whether the development of any of these agents is commercially viable in the presence of a limited market and governmental safety hurdles remains to be seen. Because contrast media are not required to provide tissue characterization, and because MRI does not produce even the very slight tissue ionization of CT, it is, by comparison, "super safe."

Absence of Ionizing Radiation

The safety of MRI versus CT scanning is demonstrated in development laboratories where technical personnel commonly use their own bodies as a phantom to test a scanner, perhaps hundreds of times. (We know of two volunteers, each of whom has been scanned more than 300 times.) In clinical practice, one would not hesitate to do as many MRI scans as indicated. No prudent person would use his own body repeatedly as a CT phantom because of the cumulative effects of ionizing radiation; an inanimate phantom is invariably used in CT. (To our knowledge, the maximum number of CT scans in any one patient is 29.)

Tissue Heating

Because MRI does not use X-rays, there is no possibility of tissue ionization; but another effect—tissue heating—occurs to some degree. This is due partly to rapidly changing gradient fields, but mostly to radio-frequency excitation energy. Only a very small fraction of the radio-frequency energy pumped into the tissues is absorbed by resonant nuclei; most of the absorbed energy simply sets up currents in the tissue, thus generating heat.

Particularly for body scans of heavy patients, much power is required to produce 90° pulses and, especially, 180° pulses. It is largely concern over tissue heating that limits the elaboration of pulse sequences and the tissue characterization obtained from them: The number of radio-frequency pulses that can be transmitted into the tissues per unit time is limited. The main field strength of a scanner is a factor: with high field strength machines, stronger excitation pulses are needed, and tissue heating is correspondingly greater.

In summary, MRI seems to be the most versatile imaging probe yet introduced into medicine. It has an unprecedented ability to characterize tissues, and it appears to be entirely harmless.

LIMITATIONS OF MRI

At the present time, MRI has several limitations: (1) complexity and high cost, (2) long scan time, (3) audible noise, (4) isolation of patient, and (5) exclusion of patients with pacemakers and metallic artifacts. The most important consequence of these limitations is that a substantial percentage of in-hospital patients cannot be scanned by MRI. Three of these problems—long scan time, confinement, and noise—cause enough patient discomfort that only cooperative and alert patients can be scanned successively. These problems are being researched, and will undoubtedly be designed out of future MRI scanners. But problems with pacemakers and metallic artifacts are more intractable.

Gantry Size and Confinement

Superficially, the MRI gantry looks like a CT gantry, because both have cylindrical patient spaces. But upon closer inspection, we can see that the MRI gantry is quite different. The most obvious difference is in the depth of the patient space. In most MRI systems, which use resistive or superconductive magnets, the patient space is much longer than that of the CT scanner. In an MRI scanner, the patient space is on the order of two meters; its diameter is one-half to one-third its length (Figure 9–4).

The dimensions of the gantry are dictated by the size and placement of the several coils needed to produce the magnetic fields used in MRI imaging. The size and shape of the gantry opening is important in patient management, because the anatomical region to be examined must occupy the center of this cylindrical volume. Particularly if the region being imaged is the head, the patient may experience a considerable sense of isolation. After a long period of confinement, totalling perhaps an hour, a substantial number of patients become significantly anxious and claustrophobic. Occasionally, patients will look at the deep space in which they are to be confined

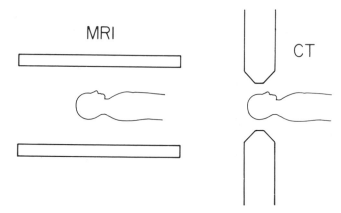

FIG. 9–4. In a CT scanner (*right*), the patient experiences little discomfort, due to the shallow gantry, low noise, and short scan time. In an MRI scanner (*left*) the patient is placed in a long cylinder. A sense of confinement is exacerbated by the loud machine-gun-like noise, and long scan time.

and refuse to be placed in scanning position. The isolation also makes it difficult to monitor the ill patient, who could experience vomiting, respiratory distress, or unnoticed movement, in addition to the emotional reactions discussed above.

No ferromagnetic support apparatus, such as tanks of gas, can be allowed inside the gantry opening since they would distort the field, ruining the necessary field homogeneity; they might even be pulled from the patient by the scanner's magnetic field. Fortunately, most modern venous infusion apparatus, pharyngeal airways, etc., are made of plastic and aluminum and so do not interact with the field. One scanner being marketed by Toshiba-America is called "Access" because the scanner is designed to allow free access to all regions of the body during scanning.

Long Scan Time

In 1990, the usual scan period during which the subject must remain immobile was between about 5 and 15 minutes. At present, this is the most limiting of the disadvantages of magnetic imaging. The throughput of patients (the number that can be examined per day) is considerably less than with CT.

Why is the scan time so long? As discussed in Chapter 5, in MRI the tissues are exposed to brief pulses of radio-frequency energy, a few milliseconds in length, resulting in stimulation of hydrogen nuclei. A substantial period of time (0.5–2.0 seconds) must be allowed to pass in order for the nuclei to dissipate their energy, and for the tissue to again be receptive to the energy in the next pulse. In most MRI imaging, the tissues are stimulated by a sequence of pulses, rather than just a single pulse (Chapter 6). The tissues are exposed to a staccato burst of several radio-frequency pulses. The series of stimulating pulses, and the subsequent re-emitted signals and echoes from which T_2-weighted MRI scans are reconstructed, occur in a period of about 100 milliseconds. After a pause of perhaps 0.5–2.0 seconds, the series of pulses is repeated. This waiting period must be provided to allow the nuclei to relax to the resting, low-energy state they possessed before stimulation (Figure 9–5). Most of the time spent in the imaging of a single slice of tissue is dead time, during which the nuclei are "cooling off." For this reason, MRI scanning is quite lengthy.

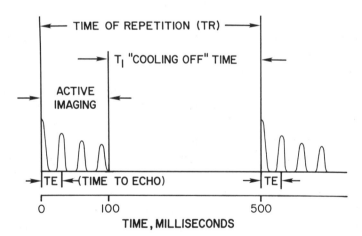

FIG. 9–5. Most of the information from which an MRI scan is reconstructed is contained in the series of echoes that occur within the 100 milliseconds of a pulse-sequence. Most imaging uses repeated pulse-sequences; before the sequence can be repeated, a considerable amount of time is required to allow T_1 energy loss ("cooling off" time). This greatly lengthens scan time.

One approach that has been taken to shortening scan time has been *multi-slice* imaging. Instead of completing the imaging of one slice of tissue before moving on to the next slice, modern scanners image several adjacent slices in the same scan sequence. By using appropriate excitation frequencies, adjacent slices are stimulated in rapid sequence; while previously excited slices are cooling off, the scanner is stimulating the next slice. By the time the scanner has finished stimulating the last slice, the first slice has returned to its pre-stimulation state, and can again be stimulated. Multi-slice techniques were a major advance in shortening scan time. Using multi-slice imaging, up to 15 adjacent slices of tissue can be imaged in the amount of time it previously took to image one.

Another approach, which produces images of lower quality in a very short period of time (a few seconds) is called *flash scanning*. In this technique, low energy pulses, which tip the magnetization vector only 10°–20°, degrees, are applied in rapid sequence, with a time of repetition (TR) of perhaps 10–50 milliseconds.

Gradient Coil Noise

Any conductive metal, when immersed in a magnetic field, is subjected to a force when electric current passes through it. This is the basis of electric motors and audio loudspeakers. In the latter, the intermittent electric current results in movement of the voice coil and speaker cone, with the consequent production of sound.

The gradient coils, housed within the gantry of the MRI scanner, lie within the larger main field coils and so are subjected to the intense main field. In order to generate the gradient magnetic fields needed for imaging, electric current must be passed through the gradient coils. This electron current interacts with the main field, causing a physical force to be applied to the coil. The electric current is passed through the gradient coils intermittently; each time the current is started or stopped, the coils are displaced slightly, but abruptly, producing a sharp sound. Because, with multi-slice excitation, the gradients must be turned on and off many times per second, a machine-gun-like noise is produced, which in some scanners can reach an 80–90 decibel sound level. This is louder than the noise in an automobile travelling at 100 kilometers per hour with the windows open.

Patient Discomfort

We can better appreciate patient discomfort if we look at it from the patient's perspective. First, patients are passed through a metal detector and placed on a hard bed. Then, they are pushed into a narrow tunnel until they come to rest deep inside the machine. They are told to remain immobile and that there will be a loud noise while they are actually being examined. Although there is voice communication via an intercom to the operator, the patients do not hear anyone physically present in the room with them. After about 15 minutes of isolation, the machine-gun-like noise stops, and a voice tells them to relax. After perhaps 2–3 minutes, the original instructions are repeated and another 15 minute period of noise is endured. If all has gone well and the scan is satisfactory, they are pulled out of the tunnel and released.

To endure this long, noisy confinement, without moving, requires a cooperative patient with considerable self-control. If the patient is in pain, has a short attention span or obstructed respiration, or for any other reason has to move, he is not suitable for scanning by current MRI scanners. This restriction may involve a substantial percentage of hospitalized patients. Undoubtedly, with further hardware and software development, scan times will be significantly shortened and the gradient coil noise muffled.

CT scanning, on the other hand, requires immobility (in a relatively unconfined space) for only 2–10 seconds per slice. The CT scanner itself is virtually silent; almost all patients can be examined for the needed series of scans. As with MRI, patients are not aware of the actual interaction of the diagnostic probe with their bodies.

Pacemakers

A cardiac pacemaker consists of a small electronic package surgically implanted under the skin, high on the right anterior chest wall, with stimulating wires extending into the subclavian vein and, ultimately, into the apex of the right ventricle. These devices usually are of the "demand" type, triggering heart action only after a pre-set period of electrical silence (a few seconds); a pacemaker may fire only rarely. To test its viability, a magnetically sensitive switch is included in the device; this switch may be activated by a permanent magnet placed on the skin over the pacemaker, which responds by creating a preset regular heart rhythm. This is a routine test procedure performed by the patient's cardiologist.

Given this situation, it seems unwise to place a patient with a pacemaker into the main field of an MRI scanner, since this will start the pacemaker's regular rhythm. This probably is harmless in most circumstances, even though the patient may be in a scanner for as long as an hour. Nevertheless, placing the patient in the field tampers with this vital device and, at present, most physicians avoid scanning patients known to have a pacemaker. We have learned informally that several patients with pacemakers have been inadvertently scanned, with no apparent ill effect. Future pacemakers will probably be designed to be insensitive to external magnetic fields and radio-frequency pulses.

Tissue Metal Artifacts

For successful imaging to take place, the magnetic field of the MRI scanner must be highly uniform. Metals imbedded in tissues can present a problem in MRI if they are ferromagnetic. Such metals are attracted to magnets; they also concentrate (and thus distort) the magnetic field. Iron and some types of steel are the most common ferromagnetic materials encountered in MRI.

When a piece of iron-steel appears in the MRI scanner's field, it creates two problems. First, it concentrates the magnetic lines of force of the main field, causing a regional loss of homogeneity. A piece of steel only a few millimeters in diameter (shrapnel, for example) may effectively erase the image over several centimeters in all directions. This is unlike CT, in which image artifacts are confined to only those sections in which the metal lies, adjacent sections being completely unaffected. In MRI, a significant regional artifact may be caused by a piece of iron so small as to require radiography to identify its location. An additional problem is that the magnetic field of the scanner exerts a force upon the ferromagnetic metal. Near the opening at either end of the scanner, there is a rapid convergence of the field, causing very steep gradients. Any ferromagnetic material brought into this region will be forcefully attracted into the magnet. Although this is a potential problem with iron imbedded in the body, it is more often a problem with large objects such as tanks of gas or wrenches. Such objects can be accelerated so abruptly that this phenomenon is called the *missile effect*. In one case report, an unrecognized small piece of steel in the eye of the patient moved upon entering an MRI scanner, resulting in hemorrhage and visual impairment (Kelly et al., 1986).

When elongated iron structures are subjected to a magnetic field, they tend to align themselves with the field and generate a torque, much as a compass needle aligning with the earth's field. This torque is much stronger than that experienced by a compass needle, however, since the MRI scanner's field can be 20,000–30,000 times stronger than the earth's field. This could be a source of danger in patients having ferromagnetic clips on blood vessels. Although this effect has been the subject of much speculation, there has been no published report of injury. Future vascular clips should not be ferromagnetic.

Fortunately, most metals implanted surgically are not significantly ferromagnetic. All steels are mostly iron, but high-nickel-content steels (over about 15% nickel) are very weakly ferromagnetic. Dental fillings of mercury-silver amalgam or gold are not at all ferromagnetic. Similarly, tantalum, silver, copper, plastics, lead bullets, and other materials commonly implanted in the body are not ferromagnetic. (See reviews by Paul New, 1983.) MRI ignores most metals: they appear as voids, as does bone.

Metal detectors (like those used in airports) at the entrances of the room housing the MRI scanner are now routine, but they sense only fairly large objects. Vascular clips cannot be detected other than by radiography. When there is any doubt (caused by the presence of a surgical scar, or a history of previous major surgery), a radiograph of the operative area will establish the presence of tissue metal artifacts. It cannot, however, determine whether they are ferromagnetic.

Complexity and Cost

MRI is the most complex technology yet applied in clinical medicine. Its predecessor, CT scanning, is perhaps an order of magnitude simpler in theory and practice. MRI hardware and physician training are accordingly more expensive. Personnel costs include the interpreting physician and at least two technical operators. As noted in Chapter 7, magnetic and electrical shielding are needed for optimal performance. These add to the site costs and tend to limit possible locations. Particularly for high-field machines, this may require locating the scanner at an inconvenient distance from other related imaging apparatus.

In view of the lower patient throughput and the much greater costs of purchase, site preparation, and hardware maintenance for the scanner, MRI procedures are accordingly more costly. A substantial reduction in manufacturing cost may result from newer superconducting ceramics, which become superconducting at temperatures above 100° kelvin. Because this is substantially above the boiling point of nitrogen, liquid nitrogen can be used for cooling. If these ceramics are shown to be practical for use in large MRI magnets, they will greatly simplify the internal structure of the magnets and obviate the need for liquid helium. In 1990, the major problem with developing this technology for use in MRI was fabricating a wire that possessed two important qualities: high reliability and the ability to carry the necessary current load. At present, "warm superconductors" lose their superconductivity when more than a trickle of current is passed through them.

10

Advantages and Limitations of CT

Computerized tomography (CT) was the first modern imaging technique, becoming commercially available in 1973. It was in use for about ten years before commercial MRI scanners began to be marketed. The success of CT stimulated the development of not only MRI, but other tomographic techniques, such as positron emission tomography (PET), and single-photon emission computerized tomography (SPECT).

CT scanning has several advantages. The most important of these is short scan time: one slice can be imaged in 1–5 seconds. Unlike MRI, the presence of ferrous metallic objects and pacemakers in the patient does not preclude scanning. For these reasons, CT is universally applicable: essentially all patients can be scanned. The exception is those who cannot remain motionless for even the short duration of the scan. In addition, both the theory and application of CT to scanning of patients are easily comprehended. Consequently CT has been, and remains, an extremely valuable diagnostic tool. However, it also has several fundamental limitations. The most important are: (1) limited tissue characterization due to the nature of the X-ray probe, (2) restriction of CT scanning to transverse slices due to physical constraints, and (3) its inability to image certain anatomical regions.

CT TISSUE CHARACTERIZATION

Specific Gravity

One might suppose that X-rays are absorbed by tissues, and that a medical radiograph is the result of this absorption. In fact, this is not true: the atoms that make up the soft tissues of the body are not efficient absorbers of diagnostic X-rays. To absorb X-rays efficiently, an atom must have a high atomic number; most of the body's tissue atoms—hydrogen, carbon, oxygen, and nitrogen— have too low an atomic number. These light atoms interact with X-rays in another manner—they deflect the X-rays away from their original path. This deflection is known as *Compton scattering*, which creates a shadow of anatomical structure (thus creating the radiographic image). But in soft tissues it also creates a random forward spray of X-rays (Figure 10–1). On a medical radiograph, this scattering fogs the film, obscuring the desired shadows of real, anatomical structure.

Rather than being a hindrance, in CT scanning the scattering of X-rays by soft tissues is essential to the creation of the image. CT uses a narrow beam of X-rays, which follow a precisely defined path between source and detector. When the X-rays are deflected from their original path (by even a small angle), they fail to strike

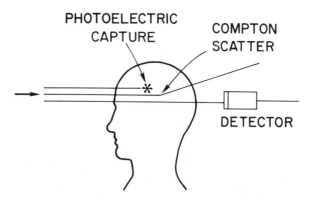

FIG. 10–1. Three X-rays enter the head in the direction of the detector. The bottom X-ray reaches the detector, since it does not interact with the tissues. The upper X-ray collides with, and loses all its energy to an atom; this photoelectric capture usually occurs with only very heavy atoms, such as iodine in contrast media. The middle X-ray undergoes a grazing collision with a tissue atom, is deflected a few degrees from its path, and misses the detector; this Compton scattering is the most common interaction between diagnostic X-rays and tissue atoms. These two types of interaction are the only sources of tissue characterization in CT.

the detector. The deflected X-ray does not fog the image reconstructed by the computer but leaves the imaging process completely, as if it had been absorbed. This contributes significantly to clarity of structural detail in CT.

Compton scattering is essentially the only type of interaction between diagnostic X-rays and tissues (in the absence of contrast media). The fact that there is only this one type of interaction means that there is only limited characterization of tissues available from CT. Because the number of X-rays undergoing Compton scattering is proportional to the total mass of tissue in the path, the CT scan is largely a regional map of the density (specific gravity) of tissues. If one had to choose a tissue characteristic for clinical diagnostic use, one would scarcely choose tissue density. But because of the nature of Compton scattering, tissue density is all that is available. This is true not only in CT but in all X-ray images, since they essentially represent the scattering of incident X-rays by the tissues being radiographed.

In the case of CT, the ability to image the regional density with considerable precision has produced anatomical correlations that clearly have been of enormous clinical usefulness. The modern CT scanner can measure tissue density to a precision of one-tenth of one percent of the density of water. This is called one Hounsfield unit.

One unique application of the ability to measure specific gravity has been the calculation of the brain's net weight during life. In the cranial cavity, the living brain is almost weightless, being buoyed up almost completely by cerebrospinal fluid. Before CT, it was impossible to calculate or measure the net weight of the brain during life, and after death it was impossible to duplicate the circumstances found during life. From CT measurements, it is possible to estimate that a healthy 1,200–1,500 gram living brain has a net weight in cerebrospinal fluid of some 15–20 grams.

Iodine Distribution in Contrasted Scans

The preceding discussion refers to Compton scattering of energetic X-rays by the light atoms normally found in brain. If, however, we inject into the patient a considerable quantity of heavier atoms (such as iodine), absorption occurs and the X-ray, in effect, disappears. This adds a second source of information from CT. The iodine atom contains several shells of orbiting electrons. When an X-ray passes through the atom, it can transfer its entire energy to one of the tightly bound inner K-shell electrons. The electron is driven out of the atom and comes to rest nearby. Termed *photo-electric capture*, this process is the reason why, gram for gram, iodine is much more effective at deleting X-rays from the beam than is living tissue. Iodinated contrast media have been used in angiography since the late 1930s and were readily applied to CT.

Although some 40 grams of iodine is injected in contrasted CT scanning, only a very small fraction of this appears in brain, and it is normally confined to the blood passing through the brain; iodine allows the contrasted CT scan to show the distribution of blood. Contrasted scans also show regions with a defective blood-brain barrier, where the iodine has leaked out of the blood into the brain extracellular tissue space; about 20% of brain volume is extracellular fluid, so there is a substantial anatomical compartment into which iodine can disperse.

The contrasted scan is a composite of the uncontrasted map (from the scattering of X-rays by soft tissue atoms), onto which is superimposed the distribution of the injected iodine. On the contrasted CT image, blood in large vessels becomes much brighter; non-neural tissues become generally brighter as the iodine distributes into their blood content and into interstitial extracellular fluid. Since the iodinated contrast agents are excreted by renal glomerular filtration, the iodine content of the renal medulla and urinary outflow tract rises quickly. In healthy brain tissues, iodine remains confined to blood; it does not distribute to brain tissue because of the blood-brain barrier.

In the uncontrasted scan, the image of density can be obtained without discomfort or hazard, but with the introduction of iodine the procedure is converted from harmless to mildly invasive.

The Role of the Blood-Brain Barrier in Contrasted Scans

The capillaries of non-neural tissues are permeable: there is free exchange between capillary and interstitial extracellular fluid of all substances with a lower molecular weight. This occurs because of the gaps between the endothelial cells that make up the capillary wall; these gaps are large enough to allow most molecules and large proteins to pass freely. But in brain and spinal cord, the walls of the capillaries are structured differently. Because of their unique structure, they are only selectively permeable; different classes of compounds cross the capillary at widely differing rates. This selective permeability is termed the *blood-brain barrier* (BBB).

To most charged molecules, the brain capillaries are extremely impermeable. Most modern water soluble contrast media are salts, and thus are electrically charged in solution. As a result, in healthy brain, contrast material cannot cross the blood-brain barrier and is confined to blood; this allows some of the larger vessels to be imaged clearly. The entire brain, but especially gray matter (with its greater blood volume) lightens perceptibly as the iodine distributes throughout the body in the first 30–60 seconds after injection. In regions of brain that are abnormal for any reason (tumor, trauma, etc.), the brain cannot maintain its blood-brain barrier. In these lesions, iodine leaks through the now-permeable capillaries and achieves a high regional tissue concentration. Consequently, the lesion brightens visibly against the relatively dark background of the surrounding healthy brain.

For the benefit of readers with a background in nuclear medicine, the contrasted CT scan can also be compared to a radionuclide scan. In radionuclide scanning, pertechnetate ion ($^{99m}TcO_4^-$), which has been in use since 1964, is injected into the patient. The pertechnetate ion distributes in much the same way as iodinated contrast media. The unstable Tc^{99m} decays, producing a gamma ray, which is detected by an array of detectors surrounding the patient's head. The radionuclide scan, formed by the detection of these gamma rays, is an image of pertechnetate ion distribution. (The resolution of the radionuclide scan is much lower than that of CT or MRI.) Because pertechnetate ion distributes in a manner very similar to iodinated contrast media, the information contained in the radionuclide scan is, in principle, the same as the information added to the CT scan by injecting contrast media. To summarize: Supplementing the CT scan by injecting contrast medium superimposes on the uncontrasted CT scan an image that is very similar to the radionuclide scan, but of much higher spatial resolution.

The Need for Contrast Injection

In the very early days of CT scanning, the resolution was so poor (an 80×80 display matrix was used) and statistically noisy, that extra enhancement was needed to visualize lesions. This was obtained by injecting the patient with a large intravenous dose of iodinated contrast material. The defective blood-brain barrier and increased blood content in various lesions (notably tumors) caused them to become much more visible than on the uncontrasted scan.

CT image quality improved throughout the 1970s. (It has been essentially constant since about 1982.) So much more detail was visible on the uncontrasted scan that it became rare to find a lesion on a contrasted scan when the uncontrasted scan had been entirely normal. Unfortunately, the practice of routinely contrasting patients was already firmly established, even though the need for it had largely passed. It remains commonplace to inject all patients being scanned unless there is a known previous reaction to iodides, or there is patient objection. A decision to use contrast medium should be made only after viewing the uncontrasted scan; if this procedure were followed, many fewer patients would be contrasted.

The generally accepted death rate from modern intravenous contrast agents is of the order of one death in 15,000–20,000 injected patients. Although this seems an "acceptably" low risk, contrast injection converts the CT scan from a completely innocuous procedure to one in which all injected patients are made briefly uncomfortable, about one in 1,000 become seriously transiently ill, and about one in 15,000–20,000 die. From a calculation of the number of CT scans done in the past 16 years, and the proportion of patients receiving contrast injection, it can be estimated that there have been more than 2,000 deaths in the United States alone from CT contrast injection. But they occur so rarely that no one institution is likely to accumulate a significant number of deaths. As a result, deaths from CT are very much under-reported in the routine medical literature. This estimate points out the need for a conservative approach to contrast agents, restricting their use to those patients who are seriously suspected of actual brain pathology, as determined from their clinical history, examination, and review of the uncontrasted scan.

In a conservative laboratory, about 25% of patients scanned would receive contrast.

Summary of CT Tissue Characterization

The two interactions between X-rays and tissue atoms—Compton scattering and photoelectric capture—are the only sources of information in CT. They give us specific gravity of the tissues and distribution of iodine, respectively. While clinically valuable, these are the only available sources of tissue characterizations, and of these two, iodine distribution requires physical invasion of the patient.

TRANSVERSE ORIENTATION OF THE CT SCAN

The orientation of the CT scan is defined by the hardware of the scanner: The X-ray source and detector are located in the gantry of the CT scanner, on opposite sides of the body. Because of these hardware limitations, CT scanning is restricted to the imaging of transverse slices of the body, although by proper positioning of the patient and tilting of the gantry, sections within perhaps 30° of transverse can also be imaged.

It is possible to create coronal or sagittal CT scans by reconstructing them from transverse images. To accomplish this, many very thin transverse sections must first be made; the computer then assembles rows of voxels from adjacent slices to create what appears to be a tissue section in a plane other than the one originally scanned. One of the disadvantages of this approach is that imaging of the many thin sections increases patient irradiation, and time of examination is greatly extended. These indirectly reconstructed odd planes are always lower in resolution than the directly scanned transverse sections from which they are made.

In an MRI scanner, however, the orientation of the cross-section is determined solely by the strength and direction of the gradient fields within the scanner. Manipulation of these gradients is accomplished electronically, without moving parts, with the consequence that MRI can image in any plane desired. The ability of MRI to create images of equally good resolution in any plane is an enormous advantage.

ANATOMICAL REGIONS INACCESSIBLE TO CT

In imaging, it is the soft tissues that are generally of interest, so CT is most useful in regions in which the volume of soft tissue is large relative to bone, and the thickness of surrounding bone is uniform. In these regions, the CT X-ray beam passes through only a minimal amount of bone, so the effect of soft tissues on the beam is maximized, and their image correspondingly improved.

Because the cranial part of the skull is relatively uniform, CT is effective in imaging much of the brain. However, it is less useful in anatomical regions where soft tissues of interest are surrounded by much bone. In such regions, the X-ray beam must traverse a large amount of bone, and the Compton scattering by bone overwhelms that by soft tissues. If in addition the bony region is irregular, the path length of the X-ray beam in the bone may vary considerably; in such irregular regions, adjacent X-ray beam paths pass through widely varying amounts of bone. Such irregular regions project many fine but intense shadows on the CT scan. These factors interfere with the acquisition of information about soft tissue. Thus the posterior fossa, which contains the cerebellum and brain stem, shows poor brain contrast. The fourth ventricle is the most prominent structure seen consistently. Similarly, the entire spinal cord, a small structure suspended in cerebrospinal fluid, and surrounded by very irregular, bony vertebral bodies, is not well seen because of the very large differences in the amount of bone that adjacent beam paths must pass through before and after they have traversed the bony spinal canal and the spinal cord inside.

The pituitary in the sella turcica is of great clinical interest, but its usually small size and its complex bony environment make it quite inaccessible by CT. Attempts at tilting the head back sharply to make a near-coronal CT section have been largely unsatisfactory. Many patients cannot achieve or maintain the very awkward position, and the many tangential X-ray paths through the maxillary bone, teeth, and dental fillings cause prohibitive streak artifacts in the brain, particulary in the pituitary. (Similar artifacts are seen radiating from any metal that lies in the tissue section.)

The interpetrous space, occupied largely by the pons, is especially inaccessible to CT. Not only is there a great deal of dense bone laterally in the petrous portion of the temporal bone, which absorbs a large portion of the X-rays the computer needs to compute the intracranial soft tissues, but the many irregular mastoid air cells surrounded by bone cast strong shadows through the interpetrous space.

TISSUE METAL ARTIFACTS

Metallic artifacts within the body, whether ferromagnetic or not, create streak artifacts on the final scan by absorbing X-rays much more than surrounding tissues. These metallic objects may seriously interfere with CT scanning, but only if they lie within the plane under examination. Adjacent sections not containing the metallic artifact appear entirely normal. This is unlike MRI, in which a ferromagnetic object of small dimensions may obliterate an entire anatomical region in all directions from the metal. Shrapnel and other small pieces of steel will likely be present in a small percentage of patients; it is not clear how MRI can avoid this artifact. CT has a great advantage in such cases.

EVOLUTION OF CT SCANNERS

During the first decade after the introduction of the first commercial CT scanner in 1973, CT scanners underwent a number of design changes. One of the main focuses of development was reducing scan time. (Another problem in early CT scanning—poor image resolution—was mentioned earlier in this chapter, along with the use of contrast media as a solution to this problem.) First generation CT scanners, such as were originally built by EMI, Ltd., under the direction of their inventor, G.N. Hounsfield, used a single narrow X-ray beam, which was created by a single collimating hole in a sheet of lead. The X-ray beam defined a line between the X-ray source (positioned on one side of the body) and the X-ray detector (positioned on the other side of the body). To make the CT scan, the X-ray source and detector were moved simultaneously in a translational motion, so that the X-ray beam defined successive parallel lines, along which measurements were taken. Then the X-ray source-detector assembly was rotated, and another pass was made across the tissue slice from a slightly different angle, defining another set of parallel lines. This was *translate-rotate* CT scanning.

In first generation scanners, long scan time was a problem, and shorter scan times were achieved by imaging two adjacent slices of tissue simultaneously. This was achieved by using a single rectangular X-ray beam, which in cross-section (in the middle of the head) was about 2.5 centimeters in height and about 2 millimeters wide. The beam was directed through the head to two detectors, each of which "saw" approximately one-half of the 2.5 centimeter length of the cross-section of the beam. By processing the signal from the two detectors separately, two adjacent 1.25-centimeter-thick slices of tissue were examined simultaneously, reducing scan time to about four minutes for each pair of slices.

Second generation scanners used approximately 30 independent beams, which fanned out from their X-ray source through a sheet of lead containing 30 collimating holes. Each of these beams was directed at its own detector. The X-ray source and detectors still moved simultaneously in a translate-rotate pattern, as in first generation scanners, but by using many more beam paths, a much larger fraction of the generated X-rays was used. The information required to create a scan was gathered faster, and this allowed scan times to be reduced from about 4 minutes (for two slices) in first generation scanners, to about 20 seconds (for one slice) in second generation scanners.

In the first and second generation CT scanners, both translation and rotation were separate motions achieved through physical displacement of X-ray source and detectors. Translational motion, in particular, was cumbersome to produce, and this kept the scan time from further shortening. Since the only requirement of CT scanning is to pass the collimated beam through the section many times from many directions, translational motion was unnecessary and was eliminated in later scanners, which used a single broad beam and many hundreds of detectors. The different beam paths required were

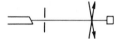

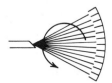

SINGLE BEAM
ROTATE-TRANSLATE
I st GENER

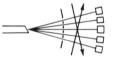

MULTIPLE BEAM
ROTATE-TRANSLATE
2nd GENER

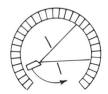

ALL ROTATE
NO TRANSLATION
3rd GENER

MULTIPLE STATIONARY
CRYSTALS
MOVING X-RAY TUBE
4th GENER

FIG. 10–2. As the design of CT scanners evolved, the relation of the X-ray source to the detector was changed. In first and second generation scanners, both the source and detector moved in translational, as well as rotational motion. In third generation, the translational motion was eliminated; both source and detectors revolved about the patient. In fourth generation, detectors were fixed and only the source moved.

created simply by rotation. In third generation scanners, both source and detectors revolve about the patient; in fourth generation scanners, only the source moves (Figure 10–2). In modern CT scanners, scan times are between 1 and 5 seconds.

It might easily be inferred that fourth generation CT scanners are superior to third generation scanners, but both types of scanners are marketed simultaneously and differences in images are not discernible.

PRACTICAL LIMITATIONS OF CT

By 1985, development of CT scanners had virtually ceased; there was no obvious direction in which to proceed. Scan times were down to a few seconds, and image processing was so fast relative to patient handling times, that no further advance seemed worthwhile. Resolution was better than 0.5 millimeters for bone/water contrast, and this is probably the practical limit of any clinical scanning method, due to inevitable patient movement from heart action, respiration, and involuntary movements.

Ironically, the X-ray tube itself, which in principle has not changed since the time of Roentgen, remains the weak link in modern CT scanners. To produce a short scan time, many X-rays must be produced per unit time. This requires very high beam currents, which push anode heat dissipation to extremes. It is common to replace two or three X-ray tubes per year. These are only partially covered by machine warranty, and not at all by service contract. After the warranty period, each X-ray tube replacement can be expected to cost $15,000–$20,000, and to result in about one day of downtime. It is not always possible to predict when X-ray tube failure will occur.

THE FUTURE OF CT

Despite these limitations, CT has revolutionized the clinical diagnosis and management of head trauma, subdural hematoma, brain atrophy, strokes (particularly with hemorrhagic components) and many other focal and general neurological diseases. Because both CT and MRI have several unique limitations at present, they will usefully complement each other, at least for a time. Because of the safety and extended tissue characterization possible with MRI, there should be a gradual shift toward magnetic studies and, very likely, a nearly complete replacement of X-rays for diagnostic purposes by the end of the century.

11

The Future of MRI

Despite our attempts at simplification, the reader might correctly conclude that MRI is a very complex process with many interdependent factors. This complexity is both bewildering and a source of hope and challenge. To exploit the magnetic properties of tissues for clinical imaging, extremely complex MRI scanners have been built. But the very complexity of the magnetic properties of tissues offers the possibility of many diagnostic strategies. In the next decade, we can expect major changes in both the hardware of the MRI scanner and the diagnostic strategies it employs.

SOFTWARE AND PULSE-SEQUENCING

The use of pulse-sequencing in MRI offers the possibility of developing many diagnostic strategies. The variables that can be adjusted in designing a pulse-sequence can be compared to the pieces and moves of a chess game: because there are many different types of chess men, each with its unique moves, there are many strategies that can be developed in a game of chess. Similarly, in MRI, there are a number of variables (pulse strength, interpulse interval, repetition times, etc.) that can be adjusted in developing pulse-sequences. New pulse-sequences are constantly being developed.

We mentioned several tissue characteristics already being exploited by MRI pulse-sequencing: hydrogen concentration, T_1 and T_2 relaxation times, and imaging of moving blood. It is possible that angiography by present invasive means ultimately will be supplanted by MRI. This will apply not only to brain vasculature but to coronary and other arteries as well. MRI's ability to image bone marrow may lead to the development of regional bone marrow imaging. Recently, MRI has also been used to image regional tissue magnetic susceptibility—the ability of tissues to concentrate magnetic fields.

When considering the future development of MRI, it is important to remember that, once the scanner hardware (main magnet, gradient coils, excitation and receiving coils, and a powerful computer) is in place, much developmental work can be done by altering the computer software, to vary pulse-sequences, gradient switching, etc. Because this can be accomplished by designing new software, without the need for new hardware, the rate of scanner obsolescence should be slower with MRI than has been the case with CT.

HARDWARE TRENDS—MAIN MAGNETS

For clinical MRI scanners, there probably will be a trend toward much lower field strengths, perhaps generated by permanent magnets. The low cost, lack of maintenance, trivial fringe field, and small site requirement of low-field MRI scanners may create a market for these scanners in applications where only ordinary tissue imaging is required.

In the mid-1980s there was a trend toward high-field (1–2 tesla) scanners; much of the trend was justified on the basis of chemical shift spectroscopy, which requires the strongest feasible field. Chemical shift spectroscopy can be performed on magnetic nuclei of elements other than hydrogen, but this is more difficult, for two reasons: elements other than hydrogen have tissue concentrations many orders of magnitude lower than hydrogen; second, they are much less efficient resonators than hydrogen, and consequently produce less signal. For example, natural fluorine resonates with about 80% of the efficiency of hydrogen. About 23 grams of fluorine in free solution would be required to generate the same signal as one gram of hydrogen. (Under normal circumstances, the concentration of flourine in soft tissues is immeasurably low.)

The problem of analyzing non-hydrogen magnetic nuclei is a more difficult problem than might at first be thought. To create sharp spectral peaks of these nuclei, they must be part of a solute in free solution, able to undergo relatively free thermal motion. If the solute is part of, or attached to, a membrane or large molecule, it is not freely moving, but is in a relatively fixed orientation to other nearby nuclei. This creates large variations in local field strength and very rapid dephasing. As a result, T_2 is greatly shortened. (See Chapter 5 for discussion of thermal motion and tissue characterizaton.)

THE ROLE OF SOLUTE MOBILITY IN IMAGING

In order for a nucleus to be imaged, it must be part of a molecule that is in solution and freely mobile. Many tissue solutes of biological interest are not freely mobile in tissues, while others of little interest possess a high degree of mobility. In brain, for example, the hydrogen spectral peak of water is very much greater than the peaks of any other nuclei. If this peak is sufficiently suppressed, other small hydrogen peaks, from hydrogen in other molecules, begin to appear. The largest of these peaks is from hydrogen in N-acetyl aspartate. Other weaker but recognizable peaks are from creatine, choline, and sometimes lactate. (For a brief explanation of MRI spectroscopy, see "Chemical Shift Spectroscopy," Chapter 7, on page 136.)

A derivative of aspartic acid, N-acetyl aspartate has long been recognized as one of the commonest small molecules in brain, accounting for 0.1% of brain net weight. It is found only in neurons, but it garnered little interest because it has little, if any, effect on neural activity. The N-acetyl derivative appears to remain in free solution because it lacks the alpha-amino acid configuration of natural amino acids that amino acid receptors need for recognition and attachment. In addition, the acetyl group also prevents the molecule from forming peptide bonds to enter into protein synthesis. Probably because of its resultant mobility, N-acetyl aspartate produces an NMR spectral peak, which is seen prominently in MRI spectroscopy.*

If deacetylated, the residual aspartate is an excitatory amino acid and cannot be imaged by MRI spectroscopy. The inability to image

---

*One would not choose N-acetyl aspartate as the subject of research, because it has no known functions, but it does appear to be mobile in solution and is easily measured in brain.

aspartate presumably correlates with some aspects of the amino acid's biological activity, such as attachment to aspartate receptors imbedded in cell membranes or with incorporation into protein molecules. These attachments presumably immobilize the aspartate, making it invisible to high resolution spectroscopy.

It is possible that a general relationship exists between the sharpness of a substance's NMR spectral peaks and its biological activity; in order for a solute to enter into the macromolecule-membrane world of metabolism, the substance may have to anchor itself to some large immobile structure and, in the process, become invisible to MRI spectroscopy.

CONCLUSIONS

The field of clinical neurology has seen many techniques that harmlessly provided information about the state of the brain's structure (Figure 11–1). Although current MRI scanners are master-

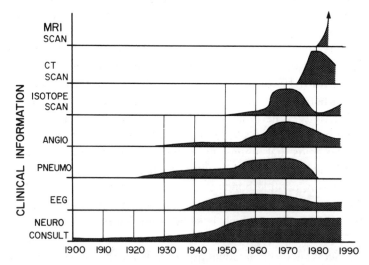

FIG. 11–1. The contribution to neurological patient management of each of several diagnostic modalities 1900–1990 is shown. The introduction of CT in the early 1970s had a significant impact on most of these tests. By the late 1970s, the active development of CT leveled off, and subsequently declined. This coincided with increased development of MRI, which has been growing at an exponential rate, indicated by the *vertical arrow*.

pieces of engineering and computer science, they undoubtedly are crude by standards that will prevail even a decade from now. The literature in this field has grown enormously in size and diversity since 1980. Many intelligent and resourceful people have recognized the power of MRI in living tissue imaging and chemical analysis.

Modern commercial firms have brought MRI a long way in just a few years. If we could direct to MRI the full force of technology and money that is now directed toward redundant war weapons and to exploration of outer space, there would be no limit to what we could learn about our own "inner space."

Appendix: An Introduction to Quantum Process in MRI

Our observation of the everyday world seems to indicate that processes such as movement and transfer of energy take place smoothly and continuously. But in the extremely small dimensions of the atom, no continuous processes occur. Atoms are about one ten-millionth of a millimeter in diameter, and a hydrogen nucleus is 100,000 times smaller than an entire atom. These are too small to be thought of intuitively and can be described only by the abstractions of quantum physics. There are no real-world objects or processes with which to compare the atoms and, especially, the much smaller nucleus.

In the world of the atomic nucleus, changes in energy content take place in discrete (quantum) steps rather than as smooth processes. The smoothly changing processes we observe in everyday life are illusions, the result of many smaller discrete quantized processes that, taken together, make up the familiar processes.

MOTION PICTURES—A QUANTIZED PROCESS

In our childhood, we were all exposed to movies, in which people and objects moved about apparently as they do in real life. At some time in our development, we learned the reality of moving pictures: that the things on the screen are not actually moving, but are only a series of nearly identical pictures flashed on the screen in such rapid succession that they appear to move smoothly. The disillusionment with what our senses tell us is roughly analogous to the transition from classical newtonian physics to modern quantum physics.

ENERGY STATES OF THE HYDROGEN NUCLEUS

To describe quantum physics and integrate it with the intricacies of MRI is an exceedingly complex undertaking, and beyond the scope of this book. But as an introduction to the usual literature of MRI we should describe for the hydrogen nucleus the alignment, stimulation, and emission of energy, in the light of modern physics. We will then have a better understanding of the fundamental processes leading to magnetic images—specifically, how the the radio signal given off by the nuclei represents nuclear behavior.

Alignment in a Strong Magnetic Field

When a compass needle aligns itself in the earth's magnetic field, it comes to rest pointing directly north. In the magnetic field of the MRI scanner, individual hydrogen nuclei attempt to align themselves but cannot align perfectly, due to the property of nuclear spin. In Chapter 3, we saw how the magnetism of certain nuclei results from the property of spin possessed by atomic particles. Nuclear spin cannot be described in terms of rate of rotation, or other terms that we associate with rotation in the macroscopic world. For example, nuclear spin does not gradually slow down. Like mass, nuclear spin is a permanent characteristic of the particle. A useful mechanical analogy to explain how nuclear spin makes the nucleus magnetic describes the nucleus as rotating about an axis. Because the positive charge of the nucleus is located off the axis of rotation, the charge moves in an approximately circular path, and produces a magnetic field in a manner analogous to the circulation of electrons in a loop of wire.

The orbiting charge makes the nucleus into a magnet with a north and south pole that lie on its axis of rotation, also called its *spin axis*. The spin axis is represented in diagrams as a straight line passing through the nucleus and extending into space in both directions. Like other magnets, the nucleus attempts to align itself in a magnetic field so that its south pole seeks the external north pole. (We note, in passing, that the end of a compass needle that points at the earth's North Pole, usually marked "North," is actually the south pole of the magnetized needle.) The nucleus does not align perfectly with the field, but tilts away from perfect alignment. The spin axis undergoes a circular wobbling motion, more properly termed *precession*. Precessional motion is familiar to us as the motion of a toy top (see Figure 6–1).

In the above analogies, spin must not be confused with precession. (A toy top in the earth's gravitational field spins about its axis of rotation at a high rate; but this spin axis precesses at a much slower rate. The earth itself rotates once per day, but its precessional motion is much slower: It completes one precessional cycle about every 26,000 years.)

The oscillatory precessional motion of the nucleus in the MRI scanner's magnetic field is comparable to the swinging motion of the compass needle in the earth's field, described earlier (Chapter 2). It can be described by the number of cycles of precessional motion that the nucleus experiences in one second; this is the *Larmor frequency* (or *nuclear magnetic resonant frequency*) of the nucleus (Chapter 3). The Larmor frequency is proportional to the magnetic field strength and is the frequency at which magnetic energy can be absorbed by the nucleus.

In summary, when the compass needle aligns itself with the earth's magnetic field, it aligns itself perfectly and comes to rest, the south pole of the compass needle pointing toward the north pole of the earth. The hydrogen nucleus in the magnetic field of the MRI scanner never comes to rest, but continually precesses. Because of its precessional motion the south pole of the hydrogen nucleus cannot point directly at the north pole of the external field, but does point in that general direction.

Stimulation at the Resonant Frequency

The situation described above, with the nucleus precessing and aligned with the field of the scanner, is the *low-energy* state that the nucleus is in before stimulation. When the hydrogen nucleus is exposed to radio energy at its Larmor frequency, the phenomenon of nuclear magnetic resonance occurs: the nucleus absorbs energy.

When it absorbs sufficient energy, the nucleus is driven from its resting, or low-energy state, into the stimulated, or *high-energy* state. This corresponds to a change in the physical orientation: the nucleus flips in the magnetic field, so that its south pole now faces the south pole of the external field. It continues to precess at its Larmor frequency. The nucleus remains in this orientation with some stability, but would "prefer" to return to its low-energy state.

Emission of Energy

Having absorbed a quantum of energy, the hydrogen nucleus in watery solutions remains in its high-energy orientation for a period of time ranging up to several seconds, depending on the chemical and physical characteristics of the solution. Eventually, under the influence of the ever-changing magnetic environment of the tissues,

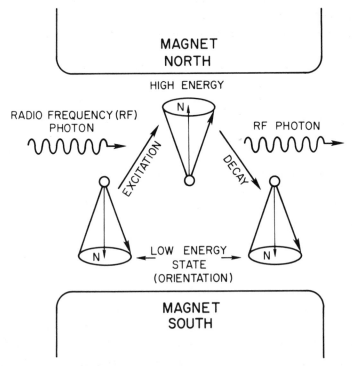

FIG. A–1. Low- and high-energy orientation. A hydrogen nucleus in its low-energy state (*left*) absorbs energy from a photon and changes orientation in the field to the high-energy state (*center*). Subsequently it decays back to the low-energy state (*right*), giving up energy as a photon.

the nucleus falls back to its low-energy state. As it does so, it re-emits its energy, the lost energy appearing as a radio-frequency photon. The nucleus returns to its original relationship to the magnetic field, its south pole directed toward the external field's north pole (Figure A–1).

Whether in the high- or low-energy state, the nucleus precesses at its Larmor frequency. The frequency of the emitted photon is the same as the Larmor frequency of the nucleus at the moment of decay. If the strength of the magnetic field has been constant throughout the cycle of stimulation and decay, the Larmor frequency remains constant, and the emitted photon has the same energy (and frequency) as the original stimulating radio wave. If, however, the strength of the magnetic field changes before the nucleus emits the proton, the frequency of the photon will change accordingly.

High- and Low-Energy States

The stimulation from low- to high-energy states, and subsequent decay from high- to low-energy states are both quantum processes. The hydrogen nucleus, with its two energy states, is unlike the compass needle, which can be deflected (stimulated) to an infinite number of angles or energy states, depending on how hard it is tapped. (Magnetic nuclei of other elements may occupy several energy states, although still only a limited number.) In this regard, the hydrogen nucleus could be compared to a domino on a table. The domino also has two energy states: lying on one flat side (its low-energy state) and standing on end (its high-energy state). To raise it from horizontal to vertical position, work must be done and energy added. When it is nudged with a horizontal force it falls, giving up (as heat and sound) precisely the amount of energy that it gained on being raised (Figure A–2). The raising and falling of the domino is a quantized process, analogous to the stimulation and decay of the hydrogen nucleus, because there are only two states the domino can occupy. The sound given off by the falling domino is somewhat analogous to the photon emitted when a nucleus falls from a high- to a low-energy state.

The difference in energy between the high- and low-energy states of the hydrogen nucleus is precisely the energy of the stimulating

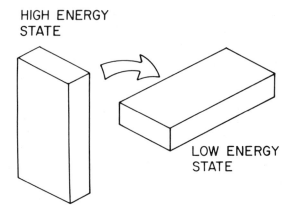

HIGH ENERGY
STATE

LOW ENERGY
STATE

FIG. A–2. Two energy states of a domino. A domino standing upright is in its high energy state. When it falls, it loses energy (as heat and sound) and comes to rest in its low energy state, lying on its side.

radio photon. The frequency of the stimulating photon is that of the Larmor frequency of the nucleus, which in turn is related to field strength. Consequently, the difference between high- and low-energy states is proportional to field strength.

Stimulated Emission

In a further extension of the domino analogy, consider the horizontal force, or "nudge," required to make the domino fall. Without this force, it would remain forever in its raised, high-energy position. The destabilizing force might come from moving the table randomly until the domino topples. The shaking table is analogous to the random magnetic forces, created by thermal motion, to which an energized nucleus is subjected. These magnetic fluctuations stimulate the emission of energy, which determines the rate of energy loss (T_1). Solids, which lack the random motion of liquids or gases are, by comparison, magnetically very quiet, and so have a very long T_1.

It is the horizontal component of the shaking table that is effective in toppling the domino. In the environment of the tissues, the direction from which the fluctuation arrives is also important: the compo-

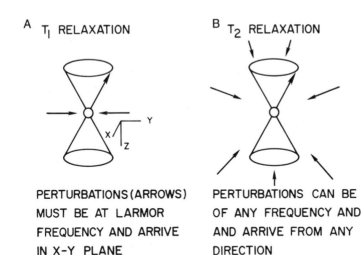

A T₁ RELAXATION

PERTURBATIONS (ARROWS)
MUST BE AT LARMOR
FREQUENCY AND ARRIVE
IN X-Y PLANE

B T₂ RELAXATION

PERTURBATIONS CAN BE
OF ANY FREQUENCY AND
AND ARRIVE FROM ANY
DIRECTION

FIG. A–3. Stimulated emission. Magnetic fluctuations from the tissue environment affect both T_1 and T_2. Fluctuations of any frequency, arriving from any direction, affect T_2 (**B**). Only fluctuations at the Larmor frequency, arriving perpendicularly to the main field, stimulate the emission of energy (T_1) from the nucleus (**A**).

nent of the magnetic fluctuation arriving perpendicular to the main field is most effective at triggering T_1 decay (Figure A–3).

CONTINUOUS SIGNAL

One might notice a major discrepancy between the compass needle analogy we originally used as a model for the hydrogen nucleus and the real nucleus we have just described. In our description of the MRI imaging process, we indicated that energy is re-emitted from the tissues in an apparently smooth manner, just as a compass needle loses its energy gradually over a period of seconds, or a bell emits sound over several seconds after being struck. This implied that an individual hydrogen nucleus emits energy in a continuous manner. But as we have just seen, an individual nucleus loses its energy in an instantaneous quantum event: the emission of a single, weak radio-wave photon. How can we reconcile the differences between the quantum nature of the hydrogen nucleus and the observed, seemingly continuous behavior of the free-induction decay over several milliseconds? The answer is threefold. First, the radio-wave photon emitted by a single nucleus is much too weak to be detected. Second, very large numbers of hydrogen nuclei are involved. Third, the nuclei emit their energy individually over a period of time.

Unlike the photon emitted by the radioactive decay of nuclei, radio-wave photons are so weak that only the combined signal of perhaps ten million photons can be detected by a radio antenna. By contrast, the gamma ray (a photon) emitted by the radioactive decay of one technetium-99m nucleus has an energy of 140,000 electron volts; one such energetic photon can be detected and measured by a gamma-ray detector. (For comparison, blue light photons are about three electron volts, red light about two; individual visible light photons can be detected using an electron multiplier, often called a photo-multiplier) (Figure A–4).

The energy of the radio-wave photon emitted by one hydrogen nucleus during MRI imaging is approximately one-millionth of one electron volt—much too weak to be detected. Any detectable radio signal must consist of the summation of phenomenal numbers of these very low-energy photons. Another consequence of their low energy is that they must all be in phase (that is, reinforcing each other) in order to be measurable at all. Visible light need not be in phase in order to be seen, because individual photons are energetic enough to create the molecular changes in our retina necessary for vision. A dark-adapted eye can see individual visible light photons.

When tissue is imaged by MRI, trillions of hydrogen nuclei are stimulated into the high-energy state. The largest number of nuclear decays—and thus the strongest signal—occurs immediately after the stimulating radio pulse. As time passes, fewer decays occur and the signal fades.

In summary, although the signal decays in an apparently smooth manner, it is actually made up of many individual, weak radiowave photons. The smoothness of the decaying signal is an illusion arising from the large number of nuclei losing their energy, much like a movie is an illusion created by many individual still pictures run rapidly in sequence.

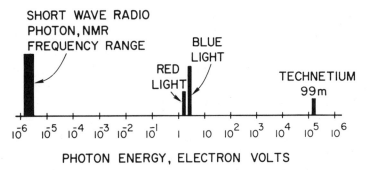

FIG. A–4. Comparison of photon energy. The energy of the radio photon emitted by the hydrogen nucleus during decay is much less than either visible light or radioactive decay. There are two consequences of this low energy: one is that a very large number of photons are required for the signal to be measurable, the other is that they must be in phase. Visible light, by comparison, need not be in phase in order to be seen; and gamma rays emitted by radioactive decay can be detected individually.

COMPARISON OF MAGNETIC NUCLEAR DECAY WITH RADIOACTIVE DECAY

In this discussion of the quantum events in MRI, the term *decay* has been used to describe the process in which energy is lost by an individual nucleus. In physics, the term *decay* is most often used to describe radioactive decay, which is both instantaneous and the photon energetic enough to be measured individually. The return to equilibrium of a large population of stimulated hydrogen nuclei over a period of time (milliseconds to hours) is referred to as *relaxation*, rather than *decay*.

The relaxation of a hydrogen nucleus during MRI has several features in common with the decay of certain radioactive isotopes. One familiar type of radioactive decay is that in which a radioactive nucleus—such as carbon-14—emits a particle and changes its atomic number or weight. In another type of radioactive decay, metastable decay, an energized nucleus emits a photon (a gamma ray) that carries away the excess energy, but the atomic number and weight remain the same.

The most common example of a nuclide that undergoes metastable decay is metastable technetium-99m (Tc^{99m}), which is widely used in nuclear medicine. (Technetium does not occur in nature, and all of its isotopes are radioactive. Since it is created artificially, it was named *technetium*.) The small *m* after *99* indicates that this nuclide is metastable: it has an excess of energy and is unstable. At some time the nucleus decays, giving up its excess energy as a photon—a gamma ray—that exits the nucleus at the speed of light, leaving it in a much more stable (low-energy) form: Tc^{99}. We can regard the metastable Tc^{99m} to be the high-energy state of the nucleus and the more stable Tc^{99} to be the low-energy form of the nucleus.

After stimulation, the hydrogen nucleus in a magnetic field has several features in common with the Tc^{99m} nucleus: it is in an unstable, high-energy state; it is also destined to undergo decay to a more stable, lower-energy state with the emission of a photon (Figure A–5). But there are major differences between the hydrogen nuclei imaged by MRI and Tc^{99m} decay. First, the photon emitted by the hydrogen nucleus during MRI can have a variable amount of energy, depending on the strength of the scanner's magnetic field. For

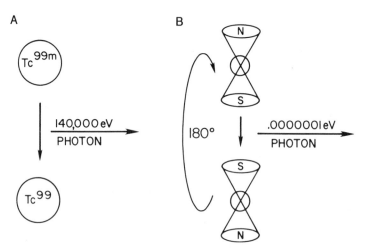

FIG. A–5. A: A metastable radioactive nuclide decays from unstable to stable states with emission of a gamma ray, without changing its atomic number or weight. **B:** Similarly, a hydrogen nucleus decays from high- to low-energy state with the emission of a radio-frequency photon, without changing its nuclear composition.

the Tc^{99m} nucleus, the energy of the emitted photon is always the same—140,000 electron volts—regardless of external conditions. Second, in MRI the rate at which emission of photons takes place varies with the strength of the field, temperature, and chemical environment. In a population of Tc^{99m}, the rate of radioactive decay (half-life) is always the same, regardless of external conditions.

COMPARISON BETWEEN RADIOACTIVE HALF-LIFE AND T_1

A further useful comparison between radioactive nuclei and hydrogen nuclei is in the terminology used to describe the rate at which they emit energy. In MRI, we have seen that, as time passes, there are fewer and fewer high-energy nuclei remaining to emit their energy: the strongest signal from the tissues is received immediately after stimulation; after that, the number of decays decreases exponentially with time. The term used to describe the rate of decay of radioactive elements is *half-life*, which is the time it takes one-half of the remaining nuclei to decay from their high- to low-energy states. Similarly, the rate at which hydrogen nuclei emit their energy after stimulation is described by the term T_1, which (for mathematical reasons) is defined as the time it takes 63% $(1-1/e)$ of the stimulated hydrogen nuclei to emit their energy. While the half-life of Tc^{99m} under all circumstances is six hours, the T_1 of hydrogen in water is variable, from milliseconds to (in solids) hours, depending on the chemical composition and physical properties of the liquid environment.

Decay of Tc^{99m} is independent of its chemical or physical environment: some circumstance inside the nucleus triggers its decay, and no means of changing it is known. T_1 decay must be stimulated by magnetic fluctuations from the external environment (from the lattice). Without such external stimulation, it might never decay.

Bibliography

BOOKS

Bradley, W. G., Adey, W. R., and Hasso, A. N. *Magnetic Resonance Imaging of the Brain, Head, and Neck.* Aspen Systems, Rockville, Maryland, 1985.

Fawcett, D. W. *The Cell.* W. B. Saunders, Philadelphia, 1981.

Farrar, T. C., Becker, E. D. *Pulse and Fourier Transform NMR.* Academic Press, New York, 1971.

Fukushima, E., and Roeder, S. B. *Experimental Pulse NMR.* Addison-Wesley, Reading, Massachusetts, 1981.

Gadian, D. G. *Nuclear Magnetic Resonance and Its Applications to Living Systems.* Clarendon Press, Oxford, 1982.

Kaufman, L., Crooks, L., Margulis, A., Eds. *Nuclear Magnetic Resonance Imaging in Medicine.* Igaku-Shoin, New York, Tokyo, 1981.

Kemp, W. *NMR in Chemistry: A Multinuclear Approach.* Macmillan, London, 1986.

Mansfield, P., and Morris, P. G. *NMR Imaging in Biomedicine.* Academic Press, New York, 1982.

Martin, M. L., Martin, G. J., and Delpeuch, *J. Practical NMR Spectroscopy.* Heyden and Son, London, 1980.

Oldendorf, W. H. *The Quest for an Image of Brain.* Raven Press, New York, 1980.

Pagels, Heinz R. *The Cosmic Code: Quantum Physics as the Language of Nature.* Pelican, Middlesex, 1984.

Partain, C. L., Price, R. R., Patton, J. A., Kulkarni, M. V., and James, A. E., Eds. *Magnetic Resonance (MR) Imaging.* Second edition. W. B. Saunders, 1987.

Valk, J., Maclean, C., and Algra, P. R. *Basic Principles of Nuclear Magnetic Resonance Imaging.* Elsevier, Amsterdam, New York, Oxford, 1985.

Young, S. W. *Nuclear Magnetic Resonance Imaging: Basic Principles.* Raven Press, New York, 1984.

ARTICLES

Bloch, F., Hanson, W., Packard, M. "Nuclear induction." *Phys. Rev.* 69: 127, 1946.

Bore, P. J., Galloway, G. J., Styles, P., Radda, G. K., Flynn, G., and Pitts, P. R. "Are quenches dangerous?" *Magnetic Resonance in Medicine* 3: 112–117, 1986.

Bottomley, P. A., Foster, T. H., Argersinger, R. E., and Pfeifer, L. M. "A review of normal tissue hydrogen NMR relaxation times and relaxation mechanisms from 1–100 MHz: Dependence on tissue type, NMR frequency, temperature, species, excision and age." *Med. Phys.* 11: 425–448, 1984.

Kelly, W. M., Paglen, P. G., Pearson, J. A., San Diego, A. G., and Soloman, M. A. "Ferromagnetism of intraocular foreign body causes unilateral blindness after MR study." *AJNR* 7: 243–245, 1986.

Lauterbur, P. C. "Image formation by induced local interactions: examples employing nuclear magnetic resonance." *Nature* 242: 5394: 190, 1973.

New, P. F., Rosen, B. R., Brady, T. J., et al. "Potential hazards and artifacts of ferromagnetic and nonferromagnetic surgical and dental materials and devices in nuclear magnetic resonance." *Radiology* 147: 139–148, 1983.

Purcell, E., Torrey, H., and Pound, R. "Resonance absorption by nuclear magnetic moments in a solid." *Phys. Rev.* 69: 37–38, 1946.

Subject Index

A

B

Blood
"black" MRI appearance of,
170–171
CT contrast scan of, 186–187
laminar flow of, 171, 172
movement of, 170–172
MRI of, 170–172
turbulence of, 171–172
Blood-brain barrier, (BBB)
contrasted scans and, 186–187
permeability of, 187
Bone
compact type, 166
invisibility in MRI, 165, 166–167
magnetic susceptibility of, 166
marrow, 154, 158, 166, 167,
195–196
in MRI interpretation, 167
in MRI scans, 156, 158, 162, 163
Brain MRI scans
cerebellar cortex in, 155
coronal section of, 156
corpus callosum of, 154
CSF and, 152, 153
gray matter of, 152, 153, 155
lesions in, 169
in neurological diagnosis, 198
pons of, 155
sagittal sections of, 154
transverse section of, 152, 153,
155, 157
T_1-weighted sequence, 152, 169

T_2-weighted sequence, 153, 169
white matter of, 152, 153

C

Chemical shift spectroscopy
of N-acetyl aspartate, 197–198
field strength requirements for,
137, 196
Larmor frequencies in, 136, 137
principles of, 136–137
signal production mobility and,
137, 197
Component vectors
dephasing and, 84–85, 89
direction of, 75–77
longitudinal, 77–78, 80–82
longitudinal-transverse comparison, 87–89
mathematical addition of, 75–76
pulse stimulation, 77
schematic of, 72, 73, 76, 81, 88,
89
signal strength and, 78–79, 82,
93–94
stimulation effects, 77–78, 80–82,
88–89
T_1 and, 77, 80–82, 88–89, 95
T_2 and, 77, 82–83, 88–89, 95
tissue characterization and, 79
transverse, 77–78, 82–83, 84–85
Computerized tomography, (CT)
advantages
metallic objects compatible,
183, 191

Computerized tomography, (CT)
    (*contd.*)
        short scan time, 183, 193
        simplicity of, 183
    analogy for, 4–5
    Compton scatter and, 184–185,
        190
    contrasted scans
        agents in, 173–174
        BBB role in, 186–187
        iodine use in, 185–186
        principles of, 185–186
        risk in, 188–189
    development of, 3–5
    evolution of, 191–193
    of head, 5–6
    image reconstruction in, 3–4, 23,
        24, 36–39
    limitations of
        in anatomical regions of soft tis-
            sue, 190–191
        Compton scatter and, 184–185,
            190
        contrast agent risk, 188
        reconstruction of image in, 189
        transverse orientation of,
            189–190
    principles of, 183, 185
    resolution in, 194
    tissue specific gravity and, 6,
        183–185
    tomography concept in, 4–5
    X-ray source in, 191–193
Computers
    in CT imaging, 36–39
    in image reconstruction, 35–39
    in MRI, 35–39
Contrast agents
    copper as, 173
    CT use of, 173
    gadolinium as, 58, 60, 173
    manganese as, 58, 60, 173
    metal chelates as, 173
    MRI use of, 58–60, 172–174
    oxygen, gaseous as, 58, 59, 60, 173
    paramagnetism and, 59–60, 173

D
Dephasing
    blood flow and, 171–172
    free-induction decay and, 99
    non-uniform magnetic field and,
        83–84
    signal strength and, 84–85, 95–96
    sources of, 83–84, 87, 99
    in spin-echo, 101–104, 106–107
    T_1 and, 89
    T_2 and, 83, 85, 87, 89
    T_2-star and, 83–84, 85, 87,
        95–96, 99, 103–104
Diagnosis
    autopsy in, 7–8
    CT scan in, 3–6
    imaging techniques in, 1–7, 198
    MRI in, 6–7, 198
    in neurology, 198
    percussion in, 2
    sensory imaging in, 1–2
    tissue environment and, 43
    X-ray in, 2–3

E

F
Free induction decay
    dephasing and, 99
    pulse-sequencing and, 91–93, 99
    tissue differences in, 109
    T_1 weighting and, 108–109
    TR and, 107–108, 109

G
Gadolinium
    as contrast agent, 58, 60, 173-
    paramagnetism and, 58, 60

H
Hydrogen nucleus
    behavior, concentration and, 41
    energy state of, 202–206,
        207–208, 210
    environment of, 41–43
    gradient effects on, 27–28, 29–33

in imaging, 15, 25, 26, 27–28, 35, 41–42, 207
Larmor frequency of, 18–19, 26, 50, 52–54, 61, 62, 203, 205
localization of, 29
magnetic environment of, 41–43, 202
magnetic properties of, 15–17, 42–43, 56–57, 69–70
magnetization vector and, 71–75
oscillation of, 70–71, 203
precession and, 70–71, 203
proton and, 16
quantum physics and, 202–208
relaxation of, 209
resonant frequencies of, 28, 29–33, 50–51, 203–204
size of, 201
solute mobility and, 197
spin axis of, 71
T_1 of, 46, 52–53, 61, 206
T_2 of, 46–47, 50–52, 61
in water, 24–26, 47–50, 53

I
Imaging
brightness in, 111–112
computer reconstruction in, 35–39
a cross-section, 26–36
in CT, 3–4, 23, 36–39
energy emission in, 207–208
Fourier trasnform in, 36
frequency analysis in, 30–33
gradient field localization, 26–36
gradient rotation in, 33–34, 38
hydrogen nucleus in, 25, 26, 27–28, 35
isolation of a tissue section in, 27–29
localization in, 29–33
magnetic gradient in, 27, 37
magnetization vector and, 75
in MRI, 23–39
pixel production in, 36
pulse sequencing and, 66–67

radio wave stimulation in, 24–26, 28–29, 42
resonant frequencies in, 28, 29–30
solute mobility and, 197–198
time constants and, 43–47, 66–67
time required for, 176–178
of transverse slice, 27–32
in uniform magnetic field, 24–26
voxels and, 23–24, 35, 75
of water, 24–26
Inversion-recovery
advantages of, 112
magnetization vector in, 112–113
pulse-sequencing in, 112–114
T_1 recovery in, 112–113
T_1 relaxation for tissues in, 113
Iron, brain MRI and, 59

J,K

L
Larmor frequency, (resonant frequency)
field strength and, 18–19, 50
of hydrogen nucleus, 18–19, 26, 50, 61, 62, 203, 205
lattice noise and, 62
magnetic noise and, 62
of magnetization vector, 75
precession and, 70–71, 82
resonant frequency and, 18–19, 50, 52–54, 90–91
thermal motion and, 50, 52–54, 61
Lattice
definition of, 62
-spin interactions, 62

M
Magnetic resonance, *see also NMR*
compass needle analogy, 9–10, 16, 18, 42–45
earth's magnetic field and, 9–10, 11, 42–43
essential elements of, 10–11
gauss and, 10, 19
instrumentation in, 13
magnet and, 9, 15, 16, 18

Magnetic resonance, *see also NMR*
(*contd.*)
   magnetic field and, 9, 16–17, 18,
      42–43, 50–51, 62, 83–84
   magnetic gradient and, 10, 21
   natural frequency and, 9–10, 12
   resonance and, 12, 13, 15, 18–19,
      50–51
   telsa and, 19
Magnetic resonance imaging, (MRI)
   advantages of
      blood movement in, 170–172
      bone invisibility in, 165,
         166–167
      contrast media use, 172–174
      CSF movement in, 172–174
      radiation, absence of, 174
      regional hydrogen concentration
         determination, 167, 172
      scan in any plane, 167
      tissue characterization ability,
         167–172
   arteriography and, 172
   contrast agent use in, 59–60
   CT imaging comparison, 36–39,
      115, 165–167, 174, 179
   future developments in, 195–199
   gantry of, 175–176
   hardware trends in, 196–197
   image brightness in, 111–112
   imaging in, 23–39
   limitations of
      complexity of, 165, 175, 182
      confinement of patient in, 165,
         175–176
      cost, 175, 182
      gradient coil noise, 178–179
      heating effects, 174–175
      long scan time, 175, 176–178,
         179
      metal interference, 180–181
      pacemaker incompatibility,
         179–180
      patient access, 175–176
   magnetic field uniformity and,
      83–84

   magnetic resonance and, 9–13
   magnetization vector in, 71–75,
      84–85
   paramagnetism and, 58–59, 168
   pulse-sequencing in, 93–95,
      152–153, 195–196
   quantum process in, 201–211
   scanners for, 117–150
   of small anatomical regions,
      148–150
   spatial resolution limits of, 140
   time required for, 175–178
   T_1 in, 46
   T_2 in, 46–47
Magnetic resonance scanners
   in chemical shift spectroscopy,
      136–137, 196
   coil placement in, 148
   description of, 117
   electromagnets of
      design of, 120–121
      field orientation in, 131, 132
      field strength of, 118–119
      principles of, 119–120
      schematic of, 119, 120
      types of, 118
   excitation coil of, 147
   field strength requirements for,
      118–119, 129, 131, 132,
      134, 135–136, 139, 196
   field uniformity in, 139–140
   flash scanners in, 178
   gantry of, 117, 120, 175–176
   gradient coils of
      function of, 140–141
      gantry positions of, 143, 144,
         147
      localization function, 145–146
      magnetic field of, 141–142
      main magnetic field effects,
         142–143
      noise production by, 178–179
      placement of, 148
      saddle coils as, 144–145
      schematic of magnetic fields of,
         142, 144, 145, 146

spatial orientation by, 147
X gradient coil, 143–147
Y gradient coil, 143–147
Z gradient coil, 143
gradient field of, 117, 118
magnetic field strength, 118, 119, 196
magnet types in, 118
main field magnets of, 118–119
permanent magnet type
  advantages/limitations of, 130, 132–133, 134
  design of, 132, 133
  field orientation in, 131–132
  field strength of, 131, 132, 134
  field uniformity in, 131
  return path of, 134
  schematic of, 130, 133
recieving coil of, 147–148
resistive magnet type
  advantages/limitations of, 123–124
  coil arrangement in, 121
  electric current requirements for, 122–123
  field uniformity in, 122, 123
  heat production in, 122–123
  schematic of, 121
saddle coils of, 144–145, 148
signal-to-noise ratio in, 135–136
strong magnetic field, advantages, 135–137
strong magnetic field, disadvantages, 137–139
superconductive magnet type
  advantages/limitations of, 126–127, 128, 129, 139
  coil configuration, 125–127
  cooling for, 124–125, 126, 127–128, 182
  design of, 125–126
  field orientation in, 131
  field strength of, 129, 139
  helium requirements for, 127–128
  quench in, 128, 139

  schematic of, 126
  temperature/electrical resistance in, 124–125
surface anatomical coils for, 148–150
Magnetic resonance imaging sample scans
of abdomen, 161
of arterio-venous malformation, 157
of bone, 156, 158, 162, 163
of bone marrow, 154, 158, 163
of brain, 152, 153, 154, 155, 156
of carotid artery, 157
of chest, 160
of CSF, 152, 153, 155
of fatty tissue, 154, 155
of gray matter, 152, 153, 155
of head, sagittal section, 154
of head, transverse section, 152, 153, 155, 157
of heart, 160
of herniated intervertebral disk, 162
of knee joint, 163
of liver tumor, 161
of muscle, 155, 159
of neck, 158
pulse sequence effects, 152–153
of spinal cord, 158, 159, 162
of spleen, 161
T_1-weighted image in, 152, 158
T_2-weighted image in, 153
of white matter, 152, 153
Magnetization vector
behavior of, 74
component vectors of, 75–83
coordinate system of, 71, 75
direction of, 75–77, 87
in inversion-recovery, 112–113
Larmor frequency and, 75
for magnetic nuclei in aggregate, 71–75
magnitude of, 75–76
pulse-stimulation of, 77–78, 86

Magnetization vector (*contd.*)
  rotating frame of reference and,
      85–87
  schematic of, 72, 73
  signal generation and, 75, 78–79,
      93
  in spin-echo, 100–102
  stimulation and, 77–78
  voxel location and, 75
Manganese
  hydrogen magnetic environment
      and, 43
  magnetic properties of, 43
  paramagnetism and, 58

N

Nuclear magnetic resonance, (NMR)
  apparatus for, 90–91
  emitted energy detection in, 20
  field strength and, 18–19, 20
  free-induction decay and, 91–92
  hydrogen nucleus and, 15–17, 26,
      56–57
  Larmor frequency and, 18–19, 26,
      90–91
  magnetic field and, 16–17, 24–26,
      83–84
  magnetic nucleus, properties of,
      18–20
  nuclides and, 17
  radio wave stimulation and,
      19–20, 24–26
  resonant frequency and, 18–19, 21
  spin and, 17, 56
  stimulation in, 19–20

O

Oxygen, paramagnetic properties of,
    58, 59, 173

P

Paramagnetism
  of blood, 58
  contrast agents and, 59–60, 173
  electron orbits and, 56–57

examples of, 57–58
  gadolinium and, 58, 60
  manganese and, 58
  MRI and, 58–59, 168
  nuclear magnetism and, 57–58
  oxygen, gaseous and, 58, 59, 173
  requirements for, 58
  time constants and, 59–60, 63
Precession
  Larmor frequency and, 70–71, 82
  magnetization vector and, 74, 87
  path of, 73
  schematic of, 71, 87
  transverse vector and, 82, 84–85,
      87
Pulse-sequencing
  factors in, 97
  free induction decay and, 91–93,
      99
  future developments in, 195–196
  imaging and, 66–67, 111–112
  inversion-recovery and, 112–114
  MRI scan effects, 152–153
  pulse, strength of, 92–94, 97
  pulse, time of, 92–93, 94, 97
  signal strength and, 92, 93–95
  single pulse and, 90–92, 96
  spin-echo, 97–111
  schematic of, 93, 94
  T_1 and, 66–67, 90, 95, 96–97
  T_2 and, 66–67, 90, 95, 96–97
  timing of, 97
  variables in, 195

R

Radioactive decay
  magnetic nuclear decay and,
      209–211
  relaxation and, 209
  T_1 comparison, 211
  of technetium-99m, 210, 211
Rotating frame of reference
  radio-pulse/tissue interactions,
      85–86

schematic of, 86, 87
transverse component and, 85–86

S

Scanners, *see MRI scanners*
Spin
 definition of, 62
 electron orbits and, 56–57
 -lattice interactions and, 62
 magnetic field and, 62
 magnetism and, 56–57, 62
 -spin interactions and, 62
Spinal cord, MRI scan
 bone and, 158, 162
 herniated intervertebral disk and,
  162
 nerve roots of, 158, 159, 162
 sagittal section, 158, 159, 162
 spinal canal of, 162
Spin-echo
 amplitude of, 111
 of brain, 104
 dephasing and, 101–104
 explanation of, 100–103
 free-induction decay in, 99,
  107–108, 111
 gradient echos and, 105
 magnetic barrier in, 99, 100
 magnetization vector in, 100–102
 origin of, 99–100
 pulse-sequence diagram, 98, 101,
  106
 response, 98–99
 sequence, common for, 103–104,
  106
 T_1 determination from, 105
 T_2 determination from, 103–104
 TR in, 105–111
 T_2-star and, 103–104
 T_1 weighting in, 108–109
 T_2 weighting in, 110–111

T

Telsa, gauss relationship, 19
Thermal motion
 illustration of, 48, 49
 Larmor frequency and, 50, 52–54
 T_1 and, 52–53
 T_2 and, 50–52
 in water, 48–54, 72
Time constant$_1$, (T_1)
 characterization of, 43–44
 definition of, 44, 46
 in inversion recovery, 113–114
 longitudinal magnetization vector
  and, 77, 80–82, 88–89
 radioactive half-life comparison,
  211
 rate of energy loss and, 80–82,
  95–96
 scan-weighted, 152, 158, 168–169
 spin-echo determination and, 105
 in tissue characterization, 109,
  168–172
 TR and, 106–107, 108–109
 weighting of, 108–109
Time constant$_2$, (T_2)
 characterization of, 44–45
 definition of, 44
 dephasing and, 83, 87, 99, 103
 determination of, 103–104
 relaxation times and, 95–96, 169
 scan-weighted, 153, 168–169
 spin-echo and, 103–104
 in tissue characterization, 167–169
 TR and, 106
 tranverse magnetization vector
  and, 77, 82–83, 87, 88–89
 T_2-star and, 83–84, 87, 88–89,
  95–96, 99, 103–104
Time constants
 accuracy of, 65–66
 component vectors and, 87–89
 dephasing and, 44–45, 46, 89, 95
 energy loss rate and, 45–46,
  206–207
 factors influencing, 47–60
 of hydrogen, 46–47, 61–63
 Larmor frequency and, 61–63, 207
 in MRI, 46, 47

Time constants (*contd.*)
  paramagnetism and, 59, 61, 63
  polar macromolecules and, 54,
    55–56
  pulse-sequencing and, 66–67, 90,
    95–97
  relaxation times and, 95–96, 209
  thermal motion and, 48–56, 61, 63
  tissue compartmentation and,
    64–65
  tissue composition and, 64, 79,
    167–169
  viscosity and, 54–55
  of water, 46, 47, 48–54, 55–56,
    61–63
Time interval, (TR)
  effect of, 105–106, 111–112
  examples of, 108–111
  free-induction decay and,
    107–108, 109
  in pulse-sequencing, 97, 105–111
  T_1 and, 106–107
  tissue contrast and, 108–109
  T_1-weighting and, 108–109
Tissue characterization
  blood movement in, 170–172
  compartmentation in, 64–65
  component vectors and, 79
  composition of, 58–59, 64, 79,
    167
  by CT, 183–189
  in diagnosis, 43
  environment of hydrogen and,
    41–43
  fluid movement in, 167, 170–172
  iron effects, 59

magnetic field fluctuations and,
    47–60
microviscosity and, 54–55
oxygen and, 58, 59, 169
paramagnetism and, 56–59, 63
polar macromolecules and, 55–56,
    63
radio frequency probe and, 42
temperature and, 53–54, 63, 169
thermal motion and, 48–54
T_1, T_2 in, 43–45, 47, 50–54,
    63–65, 79, 109–110, 169
voxel of, 65
water and, 43, 46, 47, 167, 168

U

V
Voxels
  energy absorption in, 107
  illustration of, 24, 25, 35
  in imaging, 23–24, 35, 75
  position location of, 35, 75
  signal strength from, 78–79

W
Water
  Larmor frequency and, 61
  polar macromolecules and, 54,
    55–56
  temperature and, 53–54
  thermal motion and, 48–54, 61
  time constants for, 46–47
  tissue environment of, 43, 46, 47
  uniform magnetic field imaging of,
    24–26
  viscosity of, 54–55